Somet... on my mind

Kate Jowell

A battle with Alzheimer's

Sharon Sorour-Morris

M000303712

Published by Oshun Books
an imprint of Random House Struik (Pty) Ltd
Company Reg. No. 1966/003153/07
80 McKenzie Street, Cape Town, 8001
PO Box 1144, Cape Town, 8000, South Africa

www.oshunbooks.co.za

First published 2009

1 3 5 7 9 10 8 6 4 2

Publication © Oshun Books 2009
Text © Neil Jowell and Sharon Sorour-Morris 2009

Cover image © Brian Astbury

All rights reserved. No part of this publication may be reproduced,
stored in a retrieval system or transmitted, in any form or by any means,
electronic, mechanical, photocopying, recording or otherwise,
without the prior written permission of the copyright owners.

PUBLISHER: Marlene Fryer
MANAGING EDITOR: Ronel Richter-Herbert
PROOFREADER: Trish Myers Smith
COVER DESIGNER: Natascha Adendorff-Olivier
TEXT DESIGNER AND TYPESETTER: Monique Oberholzer
PRODUCTION MANAGER: Valerie Kömmer

Set in 11.5 pt on 16 pt Adobe Garamond

Printed and bound by Paarl Print, Oosterland Street, Paarl, South Africa

ISBN 978 1 77020 090 6

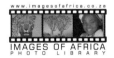

Over 50 000 unique African images available to purchase
from our image bank at www.imagesofafrica.co.za

For Kate

contents

Acknowledgements   vii

Foreword by Albie Sachs   ix

Foreword by Mike Page   xi

Foreword by Naas Steenkamp   xiii

Prologue   1

part one – EARLY YEARS   5

1   War Baby (1940–47)   7

2   African Odyssey (1947–56)   11

3   Awakening (1956–60)   16

part two – JOURNEY AWAY   21

4   London (1961–63)   23

5   *Fair Lady* (1964–66)   30

6   Love and Marriage (1966–70)   45

7   Editor (1970–72)   62

part three – A BRAIN FOR BUSINESS   77

8   MBA (1973–74)   79

9   Motherhood and More (1975–79)   89

part four – COMMANDING ATTENTION   107

    10 In Her Own Voice (1980)   109

    11 Distinguished Woman (1981–83)   125

    12 Superwoman (1983–85)   141

part five – PRIME TIME   159

    13 A Powerful Presence (1985–90)   161

    14 Down to Business (1990–93)   180

    15 In the Director's Chair (1993–99)   204

part six – AN UNCERTAIN WORLD   229

    16 Home Alone (1999–2009)   231

    Epilogue   245

    Notes   247

Acknowledgements

– To the impressive, dynamic duo at Oshun Books, Marlene Fryer and Ronel Richter-Herbert, for believing in this book and making it possible.
– To my editor, Lynda Gilfillan, for her intelligent, incisive editing, encouragement, inspiration and friendship, all of which were invaluable.
– To my husband Michael, for always being willing to read the next instalment no matter the hour, and for being gracious in his commentary, and my children, Kate Ella and Jack, for their never-ending love and hugs.
– To my parents, especially my mother, who passed away while the manuscript was in its infancy, for trusting I would get past Chapter 4!
– To John Linnegar, for his keen interest, support and excellent editing of the dreaded endnotes.
– To Paul Bowman, Lindy Smit and Patricia Swanepoel, for their very valued contribution.
– To Eunice Mzondi, for her friendship, endless cups of tea and the best rusks in Cape Town. *Enkosi kakhulu.*
– To Jane Raphaely, for introducing me to Kate and to Neil.
– To the three wise men, Albie Sachs, Mike Page and Naas Steenkamp, for their forewords, interest and involvement.
– To Neil, Justine and Nicola Jowell, for generously and warmly giving

me access to their lives at a very painful time – and for sharing Kate's story.

– Last but not least, to Kate, for taking me on this extraordinary journey. My heartfelt thanks.

Sharon Sorour-Morris

Foreword

Lucky is the person whose life story is told with grace, empathy and engaged intelligence. Unlucky is the person whose vitality is dimmed by Alzheimer's disease. This is a story of luck and un-luck. I read it with fascination. It brought back moments of a period when the movement I belonged to was being crushed, and yet I was able to snatch quiet hours of personal happiness with a bright and loving companion, Kathy Bowman, not long after to become Kate Jowell.

It reminded me of the particularity of Cape Town in the 1960s, a vivid physical setting of intense personal endeavour. Above all it memorialised a personality to whom I had been close, very close, and from whom I was to be twice separated, first by the divergence of our life itineraries, and then by her illness.

This is an intimate story of love, achievement, family and loss, a memoir without memory, reconstructed by a kind and highly literate stranger out of shards of affectionate and loving recollection. Kate appears and disappears as a protagonist herself, a living ghost that occasionally walks the ramparts of her past.

At a time when women were expected unconsciously to subordinate their minds and imaginations to those of men, Kate was vivaciously, triumphantly and overtly self-determined. Yet, the person who so successfully claimed her autonomy is now totally dependent. Her own mind that she knew so well – and that was so attractive – now eludes her. It is painful to feel that the ever-questing butterfly with darkly gilded wings has ineluctably retromorphosed into her cocoon, absent yet present at the same time.

Miraculously, the story-telling by Sharon Sorour-Morris has reconfigured her into a vital person again. What started off as a tale intended to memorialise her for close family and friends has transfigured itself through authorial charm into a richly textured and widely interesting literary portrait of one of Cape Town's most signal personalities.

So many brave women have by now shattered invisible but powerful barriers to their advance, that there is something dated about invoking 'the first woman to …' syndrome. Yet Kate truly deserves to be honoured as having been 'the first woman to …' She was the first woman to head the intensely masculine domain of the Graduate School of Business at the University of Cape Town. Viva Kate, viva! And the Business School itself becomes a major protagonist in this highly readable book.

Dedication and decency do not always lead to public success. In Kate's case, however, they did, and she used her social position and embracing feminism to make a special and distinctive contribution to the development of pragmatic social consciousness in the business community. Though, as far as I know, she never became directly involved in the underground movement against apartheid, she gave what she had to give where she was best able to give it. This was her capacity through unrelenting tactful persuasion to prepare people in her privileged circles, not only to accommodate change, but to welcome it.

The shared natural feminism of Kate Jowell and Sharon Sorour-Morris runs as a strong current right through this happy/sad tale.

For me, at least, it left a warm and poignant afterglow.

Albie Sachs
Justice of the Constitutional Court of South Africa
August 2009

Foreword

K ATE CONTINUES TO have a deep impact on my life and career. As role model, mentor and friend she displayed the character, integrity, tenacity and quiet warmth that I have always hoped to emulate. Thank you, Kate! Yours has not been a linear and narrowly focused path from student to academic, but a life journey, one that makes you unique in the best sense of the word – and you remain the most elegant person I have known.

I first met Kate when I was studying for a part-time MBA at the University of Cape Town's Graduate School of Business. Kate was on sabbatical and scheduled to teach the Industrial Relations course after the December break. Her year-long absence in no way dampened her reputation for not suffering the ill-prepared gladly. Consequently, during the break my focus was on preparing for her course, one which fully met every expectation! To me, her teaching style was superb – there was no room to hide and yet she still created an amazing and supportive learning environment. Her quick mind, wealth of experience and ability to connect classroom theory to the industrial relations challenges facing South Africa shone through.

Later, after I joined the staff and came to know her better, I was struck by Kate's generosity and quiet sense of humour. She was always willing to share her expert knowledge, general life experience and insight as an accomplished educator. This she did quite often at the King's Kitchen across the road from the old Business School campus – a diner we frequented for lunchtime toasted sandwiches and, much to her amusement, to overindulge in chocolate milkshakes, into which we asked the elderly church ladies who ran the place to deposit not one, but *two*, marshmallows.

When Kate became director of the Graduate School of Business, I worked very closely with her. We had many long brainstorming sessions to seek ways to generate the funds needed to pare down the school's debt. As always, Kate did not shirk from the huge challenge. She worked longer and harder than anybody, and never spoke badly of others, including a university administration that seemed increasingly and inappropriately to hold her accountable without providing the necessary support, particularly given its own culpability.

Some time into her term as director, with a sense of disbelief and uncertainty, I realised that all was not well with Kate. There were small clues long before the final diagnosis, but Kate showed enormous courage and was even more dedicated and hard-working in an attempt to overcome the creeping onslaught of her disease.

Knowing Kate for so many years as a vibrant, intelligent woman makes it so much sadder to see the toll that Alzheimer's is taking on a once brilliant mind. Reading this book reminded me once again of Kate's enormous successes and her impact on so many. I feel very blessed to have benefited significantly from her generous spirit. My debt of gratitude is because of her profound influence not only on my professional growth, but on the totality of my life – and how she continues to challenge me to better serve others.

With the deepest of affection and thanks.

Mike Page
Vice-president for Academic Affairs and dean of Business at the
  McCallum Graduate School, Bentley University, Massachusetts, USA
August 2009

Foreword

LUMINOUS. THAT'S THE word that always comes to mind when I think of Kate. Luminosity of mind, of person, of temperament. It is a quality that informed all she did.

One of the keys to her success was equanimity. The Kate I knew in tense board meetings was the same person as the hiker in the wilderness or the friend across the dinner table. There was an assured quietness about her that drew people to her.

One day, freshly back from a trip to Italy and France with her family, she told me about her 'little disaster'. At a petrol station restroom, she had hung her moonbag from a hook behind the door – where she had forgotten it.

'But this is not the Kate I know!' I said, because, with Kate, everything always seemed ordered. 'You'll have to get to know this one,' she said. And so I heard for the first time about the problem that had started with the inverting of digits in telephone numbers, absent-mindedness, even disorientation. The problem would become a monster that would eventually consume her life.

Living elsewhere, I was spared witnessing her decline. Then, one day, visiting her far too late, I was confronted with the shadow of what she had been. It was not only profoundly distressing. It is impossible to escape morbid fascination and its associated sense of discomfort and guilt when confronted with Alzheimer's in a person you have known well. You are in the physical presence of a departing – even departed – person. You have an intense need to relate, especially when you are facing one with whom bonds exist, bonds that are evoked by the familiarity of the face, the nuances in the now silent voice, the echoes of laughter, the things said and moments shared. You probe but find no mooring. You want to believe that you *are* relating, but you are given no means of knowing.

This is what has been experienced by those who have witnessed Kate's decline. They have been tormented by the conondrum: *Where is she?* None, I venture to say, has come to a complete and satisfying understanding.

In this sober but moving book, Sharon Sorour-Morris relates Kate's story without ever lapsing into sentimentality or undue dramatisation. The prologue tells of the Kate that she was none too long ago but no longer is; the epilogue concludes with the enigma she has become. The sixteen chapters, organised into six neat parts, tell of the influences that made her the superb, admired and well-loved person she had been, then of the first signs of the looming visitation, and finally the unrelenting decline into what now seems like a state of near-oblivion.

Sharon shares the distress of all who behold the new Kate but offers no conclusion, no moral, no solace. Yet her closing words give a certain comfort, a resigned acceptance of something you can neither change nor ever wholly understand.

We who love Kate are grateful to Sharon for telling her story so well.

Naas Steenkamp
Retired corporate executive and former member of the National
   Manpower Commission
August 2009

Prologue

IN THE VALLEY beyond, the early sun flashed sharply across the slick, indolent Vézère. The river seemed for a moment seized in its own metallic splendour. The day was glorious, summery.

The Dordogne at its best.

From her quaint hotel in riverside Montignac, the striking middle-aged woman sitting alone in the busy dining room took it all in. She contemplated the view, the bend in the river, the verdant forests. She had come on a walking tour of the pleasing White Périgord – the ancient name of the central chunk of France's famed Dordogne region – to reflect on recent, dramatic changes in her once full and demanding life.

Contemplating the day's walk ahead, she got up and crossed the room to the buffet table. She chose carefully. Cheeses, fruit, a croissant. Then she turned, plate in hand, and, at that moment, froze. Had any other guest noticed, it might have seemed that she'd paused, perhaps to select something else; that she'd suddenly remembered she'd left something at home, a telephone number, perhaps, that she'd soon be needing.

But it was nothing as familiar, or as comforting, as an oversight, or mere indecision about what to have for breakfast. At that frightening moment, she had absolutely no recollection of where she'd been sitting. She was, to all intents and purposes, lost – and it was not her Cape Town home thousands of kilometres away that she could not find, but her table, just ten paces across the room.

Kate Jowell was in the terrifying grip of Alzheimer's disease.

Three years on, the emeritus professor remembers not only the disturbing incident, but the 'desperate humiliation' of the entire trip.

'It was a terrible time. I wanted to go walking in France, and I was fit, physically. But I was not Alzheimer's fit. Every time I got up from a chair, I would not be able to find my way back to it. And when I eventually sat down, I wasn't able to turn myself to face the right way. I could have slit my throat. It was mortifying.'[1]

Her depth perception impaired by the disease, she battled to make her way down uneven and tricky declines during the walks, often needing the assistance of fellow hikers, none of whom knew of her affliction.

Yet in 2003, during our conversation, while she remembers the Dordogne debacle well, in the shifting sands of her mind nothing is really clear. She may not have visited Montignac or the White Périgord at all. It may even have been Beynac, in the Black Périgord. Frequently, simple facts elude her, and the precise details of the holiday, taken in 2000, have long been lost.

Kate Jowell was in her prime when Alzheimer's disease cruelly interrupted life as she knew it. The diagnosis of 'a progressive dementing illness' in 1999 by Cape Town neurologist Dr John Gardiner confirmed its existence. She was fifty-nine years old. But worrying symptoms had already surfaced several years before the word 'Alzheimer's' became part of her daily vocabulary.

Just two years prior to the devastating diagnosis, she was still holding office as the first woman director of the business school widely held to be South Africa's best, the University of Cape Town's Graduate School of Business. Her closest colleagues picked up worrying signs that something was wrong even then.

Kate's appointment as director in 1993 came at the pinnacle of an impressive and varied career – as women's magazine editor, academic, industrial relations fundi, business brain and mediator par excellence.

It was a career marked by firsts. In her twenties, she was one of the few women to obtain a BSc in Applied Mathematics from the University of Cape Town (UCT). Her thirties were shaped by her decision to leave the world of magazine journalism and embark on a Master of Business Administration (MBA) degree – the only woman in a class of about eighty – at her alma mater. It was to be the start of a twenty-five-year career as a lecturer at the Business School. She specialised in industrial relations, doing pioneering work, and in this time she was hand-picked to serve on high-profile government-appointed commissions to overhaul crucial labour and tax legislation. This work continued in her forties and fifties, when she was also a sought-after consultant, joining the boards of directors of top companies Sanlam, Foschini, Cadbury Schweppes, First National Bank and others.

Blessed with a quick mind, Kate Jowell was formidably intelligent. A clear thinker, she made her presence, and her opinions, felt quickly.[2] She understood business, and was confident and at ease in a man's world. She was self-contained, dedicated, hard-working. But she was also attractive and glamorous. Men found her captivating. One of her students recalls that he never heard a word she said in class, in spite of her vast teaching capabilities. 'I just kept looking at her neck – it was so beautiful!'[3]

In a career that spanned nearly thirty years, Kate Jowell became an extraordinary woman pioneer. In the 1980s, *The Star* listed her as a 'Woman of Our Time', and UCT's Commerce Faculty nominated her as its Distinguished Woman to mark the university's Centenary of Women.

Yet Kate didn't see herself as 'a spokesman for women'.[4] She didn't like the stereotype. Even so, she used every available opportunity she had 'fairly and competently' to promote women's rights and interests. Ironically, many women found her aloof, distant and intimidating, probably because of her reputation for being bright and having little time for small talk.[5]

But she had the same concerns, pressures and worries as any other woman. As a mother to daughters Justine and Nicola, and wife to leading South African businessman Neil Jowell, she juggled the demands of home with an impossibly busy working life. Once, in a radio interview, she admitted, with a self-deprecating laugh, that she managed 'poorly'. Her family contend, however, that she was highly organised and efficient.

When I meet her for our first interview in January 2003, however, Alzheimer's is taking its toll. The disease is a dementia, an affliction of the brain, and all the symptoms result from damage to the brain cells, bringing about mental and behavioural deterioration.[6] Intellectually, Kate is a shadow of her former self. The accomplished mathematician can no longer subtract seven from 100, and wouldn't even attempt the calculation. She cannot tell the time, keep track of the days of the week or write her own name.

The 'strong room' of her memory – where, in Mick Jackson's conception, we keep our life experience safe and sound[7] – has been vandalised by a relentless disease for which there is no cure. Yet, in many respects, Kate Jowell's mind is still alert and sharp. Her vast vocabulary has not yet let her down – as it almost always does in the early stages of Alzheimer's – and she is always ready with a smart retort, a witty quip.

She has coped with her decline with dignity, with humour. And while she knows she is on a dark, frightening, isolating journey, she does not easily show her distress. Her courage, under the circumstances, has been extraordinary.

This book is as much about triumph as it is about tragedy. It is an attempt to capture the indomitable spirit of an exceptional woman, to record the remarkable detail of her full life while she can still, in part, tell the story. It is an opportunity for her to reflect on it all, before, like Iris Murdoch, she 'sails into the darkness'[8] and is lost to us forever.

January 2003

part one

EARLY YEARS

War Baby

(1940–47)

I T IS IN her eyrie, the open-plan informal lounge, where I almost always find her. From here, through a vast wall of glass, Kate Jowell can track Cape Town's changing moods. The cityscape unfolds before her, with the arc of sea just beyond. The panorama is breathtaking. But Kate's favoured canvas-and-beech chair doesn't face this arresting private view. Instead, it faces inwards, towards the formal lounge.

And her eyes invariably seem fixed on the fronds of an unruly potted palm that straddles the divide between her special space and the next.

The first time I visit her, Breyten Breytenbach's *True Confessions of an Albino Terrorist* lies on the sharp-edged glass coffee table. 'I'm reading it,' she offers, 'because I'm trying to understand what it's like to be in prison.' The chilling analogy seems lost on her. In the extraordinary home that she and her husband, Neil, built in the 1980s to take in the liberating expanse of sky, sea and mountain, she is isolated, alone. Enclosed. Physically – she has not been able to drive for four years – and, most certainly, mentally. Her busy, full life and her brilliant career have been harshly pruned by Alzheimer's disease.

Her life, its story, has become a jigsaw puzzle that she can no longer piece together. But she is game to try.

'My family comes from Whitley Bay, in the North of England,' she begins, affectionately mimicking the Tyneside brogue. This piece in the puzzle is a fond certainty in her mind. But without other records and the recollection of family and friends, it would remain just a piece in an elusive whole.

In fact, Kate's beloved father was a Geordie, a man from the North. One of ten children, George William Davison Bowman was born on 9 January 1916, in Sacriston, a tiny Durham village in the heart of the coalfields. His family later moved further north, to Whitley Bay in Tyne and Wear. Life was grim. George's father was a mine captain. His mother ran the local fish-and-chips shop. The possibility of escaping the misery of mining life must certainly have seemed remote – but George was 'a brilliant guy'.[9] Even though he'd been going down the pit from the age of fourteen, he was the only sibling to obtain a Cambridge Certificate, a remarkable feat in those days, recalls Paul Bowman, Kate's older brother.

As soon as he could, George fled. He headed south, for London, where, at Mrs Peasley's Boarding House, he met the lovely Kathleen Beatrice Stone. One of the gentry whose family had fallen on hard times, Kathleen was born in Walthamstow, north-east London, on 18 September 1911.

Her father, Edward, was an abusive alcoholic who abandoned his wife and children in the 1920s. They never heard from him again. Kathleen and her four siblings – Edward, Norah, Leslie and Eileen – were raised by their mother, Madeleine, and their grandparents.

When George Bowman first came into her life, Kathleen was a carefree twenty-five-year-old working as a bookkeeper for a Bond Street jeweller in London's West End.[10] She was immediately attracted to George, with his rugged good looks, obvious intelligence and impressive resolve. Soon, the couple were madly in love and, against the odds, they married in London in 1937.

'It was during the Depression,' Paul recalls, 'and their meeting and marrying was somewhat extraordinary. There was a lot of animosity in London, as locals opposed the migration of Northerners like Dad, because they inevitably competed for the same jobs.'[11]

Kathleen's younger brother, Leslie, who also stayed at Mrs Peasley's for a while, remembers the young George as a 'dark, well-built man, with a pleasant personality'. Leslie was particularly struck by George's beautiful singing voice, and his ballroom-dancing skills. 'He courted Kathleen with the song, "I'll Take You Home Again, Kathleen". She loved it.'

The Bowmans set up home in London. The following year, on 7 May, Kathleen gave birth to their first child, Paul. George, a self-taught engineer who was very good with his hands, was earning a living as a toolmaker, but opportunities in London were limited. And so the young family relocated to the industrial city of Coventry.

It was to be a dramatic move. The world was on the cusp of war. By the time Prime Minister Neville Chamberlain told the nation on 3 September 1939 that Britain was at war with Germany, Kathleen was five months pregnant with her second child.

Leslie, who had joined the couple in Coventry, says his sister was quite resigned to it all.

'There was obviously no turning back. I remember going to visit them one Sunday morning. George was at work, as the big engineering factories worked throughout the weekend, and Kathleen started to have labour pains. She sent me to fetch the doctor, but when I got to his house the doctor's wife told me he was out. She simply shoved his black bag at me and said, "Take this!" I returned with the bag to find George at home, and Kathleen in fine fettle. It had been a false alarm.'

On 9 January 1940, Kathleen went into labour, this time for real, and gave birth to her war baby, her namesake Kathleen, who would later call herself Kathy, then Kate, 'to differentiate myself from my mother'.[12]

The chubby-cheeked baby was the apple of George's eye. Fortunately, he was not called up to fight – and nor was Leslie. 'We were both in the aircraft industry, making the parts used to build war planes like Lancasters, Spitfires, Mosquitoes,' Leslie says. 'We were in what the government called "reserved occupation" and we couldn't enlist.'[13]

But, living in Coventry, there was no escaping the reality of war. Paul Bowman can still remember the fateful night of 14 November, when one of the most devastating German bombing raids of the war left much of Coventry in smoking ruins. He was only two years old. 'I remember going into the underground shelter, hearing the bombs falling. Kate was in her crib. When it was all over and we emerged, the building that had once stood opposite our semi-detached house had been flattened.'

Both Leslie and George were keen to serve their country. Their chance came when the United States joined the war in December 1941 after Japan's unprovoked attack on Pearl Harbour. Britain's war effort was dramatically boosted and the men were free to volunteer. They joined the Royal Navy, Leslie in 1942 and George in 1944, both serving in submarines until the war ended in 1945.

Kate was five years old at the time. Almost all the photographs of her as a child show a bright-eyed little girl with a ready smile. Today her only recollection of those early years is of Paul mercilessly calling her 'fatso'.

'I used to complain to my mother, and so she suggested I call him "four-eyes", which I did!' Paul, however, simply remembers being protective of his little sister.

Post-war life in Coventry was frugal and dismal. So, in 1947, after he was demobilised, George took a passage to Africa. He was after a new beginning for himself and his family. South Africa was his first choice, but the tension and animosity he encountered on arrival in Johannesburg between English-speakers and Afrikaners put him off. He soon headed north, for Rhodesia, and fell in love with the country.

Kate had been at Earlsdon School in Coventry for some time when, aged seven, she wrote him a letter, telling him about her sweetheart Roin Youett [*sic*]. It reads, 'Dear Daddy, How are you getting on in Rhodesia? I go to Earlsdon school ... Daddy, ever since I went to Earlsdon I've had a sweet-heart, his name is Roin Youett he often tries to catch me and kiss me ... I am in Mrs Greenways class! I don't find it boring, we have knitting, we are knitting for a doll called Sally Anne ... Well ta ta and Good Luck and I hope we get the passage soon. Your loving daughter Kathleen.'

Africa beckoned.

2

African Odyssey

(1947–56)

WITH ITS BLISTERING heat, its dust and intoxicating intensity, Africa must have been a thrilling yet daunting prospect.

When Kathleen Bowman packed up her life in urban England in 1947 to follow her husband to Southern Rhodesia, where, as many believed at the time, 'Cecil John Rhodes had intended for we British to go',[14] she probably had mixed feelings. Just getting there was a challenge for a mother with two small children. As it turned out, the passage to Africa was highly eventful. Kathleen paid a huge sum for the threesome to board a Greek black-market ship bound for Mozambique.

Paul, who was nine at the time, kept a protective eye on what he saw as his two charges. 'My mother was a gorgeous woman, and the Greek crew found her very attractive and pursued her. I watched her like a hawk. I was only a little boy, but I knew what was going on!'[15]

Though seemingly interminable – the ship took four weeks to reach its destination – the voyage was fascinating.

'We went through the Suez Canal,' Paul recalls, 'and I remember seeing prisoners of war in wire enclosures. We docked at Mombasa and then Lourenço Marques.'

The unpleasant, mandatory cholera shots that preceded the voyage stand out in his memory as 'far worse than contracting the disease!'

Then there was Kate's fall. While walking on one of the upper decks, she slipped through an uncovered deck hatch and disappeared. The vessel, which carried freight as well as passengers, was crowded and 'not very organised'.[16] Fortunately, a pram on the deck below broke her fall. Paul remembers her being taken to the ship's doctor, screaming and in pain. She was not seriously injured, but the shocking incident was reported in the English papers, and was later even brought up in the House of Commons during question time.[17]

Kate's memory of the accident is vivid if impaired. 'It was a terrible thing,' she says. 'I was on the deck one minute, and the next I just slipped and fell down this hole. I think I was trying to find a toilet.'

Suddenly, as if distracted by an unexpected impulse, she veers off the topic. 'My father was so keen for us to get to Rhodesia. I wonder if that's where I lost George? I was holding him over the water and I dropped him and I thought, "That's the end of George".'[18]

Beloved George, Kate's hand-sewn toy bunny – named after her father – was an ever-willing companion and adventure seeker. And he may very well have been travelling down the east coast of Africa with Kate then. But his near demise, which Kate can't quite place, is – as gradually becomes clear to me – the subject of many other stories.

When the weary travellers disembarked at Lourenço Marques, a long train journey still awaited them. Finally reaching Bulawayo, they stepped onto what was then the longest station platform in the world for a happy reunion with George Bowman. A new life had begun.

It was exotic, exciting. But it was far from easy. The family lived in Queen's Park, in a small house made from mud. George, who could not afford a car, cycled the eight miles to and from work, morning and night. Typically, he was not discouraged. The company he worked for – Rhodesian Plough – manufactured agricultural equipment. It was not long, however, before George, an ingenious and resourceful man, left to start his own business – Bulawayo Steel Products – and he was soon joined by a young friend from Rhodesian Plough, Otto Morgenstern.

The business was a success. From its early beginnings of manufacturing components for agricultural implements the company grew to design and produce one of the first made-in-Africa ploughs, which was exported throughout the continent. But that came later.

The first years were happy, if frugal. In no time, Kathleen's brother, Leslie Stone, also felt the pull of Africa and joined the Bowmans in Bulawayo. Kate, he remembers, was 'a gorgeous child, absolutely lovely and very bright'.[19] She was conscientious, eager to please – and a born scholar. Take the revealing postscript of the letter she sent to her father in Bulawayo when she was only seven: 'P.S. Daddy, I was one of the children who went downstairs to show Miss Cole my book and she said it was very good.' Her pleasure, her excitement at being rewarded for good work, is already clearly evident.

Paul, who was to inherit his father's rugged good looks and easy charm, was very possessive of Kate when they were growing up. Once, he sternly chided a little boy who seemed to be getting rather too friendly with his sister: 'You can't have her because she's mine!'[20] Theirs was a classic 'big brother, little sister' relationship. He was proud of her, and protective. He still is.

'She was a good girl,' Paul says, 'the apple of my father's eye. He called her "Pet" and was devoted to her because she was so good, and so successful. If she got into mischief, I was mostly to blame.'

Paul's relationship with his father was trickier, though. By his own admission, he was a bit of a rebel. Kate attributes their occasional clashes to both of them 'wanting to be top dog'. Still, the family was a close-knit one. Both Kate and Paul attest to having had a happy childhood. Curiously, though, no anecdotes have emerged: there are few 'When we were young …' stories to be told. And neither Paul nor Kate can remember any special gifts they may have received – at Christmas or at any other time.

'My father was growing his company,' Kate says, 'so there was not a lot of money for presents in those early years. I don't really remember specific presents, although I'm sure my parents would have tried to do something nice. We didn't splurge, as there was not a lot of money. But there was a lot of love.'

George, the chocolate-brown toy bunny, is probably an exception. On one of my visits, she whips him out of a plastic bag, dog-eared and tired, but clearly still an object of affection. Made from fabric, and now more than fifty years old, he must have been quite natty in his day.

The incident when the toy came perilously close to disappearing from her life forever is, I soon realise, one of Kate's fixations. Every time she tells it, the story changes – sometimes slightly, often quite radically. More or less, it goes something like this: Kate and Bunny George were on a train journey *en famille*. Unable to resist the temptation, she was holding George out of the open window (probably against the good advice of her parents) when he slipped from her fingers and fell away as the train raced on. Kate's distress was such that George, her father, pleaded with the conductor to stop the train. A commotion of sorts ensued, but Bunny George was recovered, and the train resumed its insistent, rhythmic clatter to its destination.

Another object from her childhood that she shows me is her school dictionary. I arrive one day to find Kate waiting for me at the bottom of the steep staircase that takes visitors from the front door of the Jowells' Glencoe Road home to the hub of the house. She is beside herself, clutching a small, faded maroon book that she places carefully in my hands.

'Look what I've found!' she exclaims. It is her *Everyman's English Dictionary*[21] in which, in careful cursive, she'd inscribed the words 'Kathleen Bowman. Convent High School, Bulawayo. Address – 3141, 11th Ave., Queen's Park West, Bulawayo.'

Kate attended Bulawayo Convent for most of her school life. She was a model scholar – clever and diligent. Blessed with an extraordinary aptitude for mathematics – which was just as well, since her father hoped she would become a mathematician – she was one of the cleverest convent pupils in Rhodesia.[22]

'She was also a very good pianist,' Paul remembers, 'and she always did very well when she competed in eisteddfods.'

Like so much else in her life, however, Bulawayo Convent is no more. The school buildings may remain, but its once noisy playgrounds and busy classrooms are now silent.

By the time Kate matriculated, at fifteen, the Bowmans had long since moved to a more affluent Bulawayo suburb, to 17 Scott Street,

North End. Often, at weekends, Paul and Kate and a group of friends would head for the Matopos, where, among the magnificent koppies, Cecil John Rhodes lies buried.

'We'd go up with my parents, on the back of my dad's brown Austin pick-up truck, which he used for his business,' Paul says. 'We'd play cricket at the Matopos and then we'd go up into the hills to explore. It was great fun … those were good times in Rhodesia.'

The two siblings lived in Bulawayo until, within a year of each other, they left Rhodesia to discover what the world had to offer. After that, they would return only as visitors.

3

Awakening

(1956–60)

F EBRUARY 2003. A bone-chilling wind ushers us into the house.
Kate and I have been to Carlucci's, a trendy deli she often visits in
Cape Town's lush Oranjezicht suburb, to mull over events that took
place in her past.

Four years ago, when her doctor instructed her to stop driving,
she would walk the relatively short distance from Glencoe Road to
Carlucci's – for the exercise as much as for the cappuccinos. Or friends
like Yvonne Galombik, wife of the late Arnold Galombik, legendary legal
brain, Trencor legal adviser and a close family friend, would drive her
down as a treat. Now, her once sure stride is an uncertain shuffle, thanks
to 'Mr Alzheimer's' – as she often refers to her affliction – and so, she
has to be driven. Like today. It is mid-afternoon, and she's weary. After
one of my many questions, she retorts, 'I'm clueless. I'm trying to see
what I can dredge out of my mind today, but it's terribly foggy.'[23]

Back home, we're joined by Justine, the Jowells' eldest daughter, who
has come to take us through the family photograph album, put together
by her younger sister, Nicola, who is living and working in Bristol in
the United Kingdom.

'Nicola is the only one who's organised enough to put together something like this!' Justine says with a laugh.

We sit next to one another in Kate's favourite space, with its dramatic
view. Justine points to photographs in the album, picks out people and

places. Kate battles to keep up. She appears confused, disorientated. The array of photographs is intriguing. There is a photograph of the 'Capricorns' – Kate and two girlfriends, well-known journalist Gorry Bowes Taylor and former *Fair Lady* food editor Annette Kesler – all of whom have a birthday in January and have, for the past thirty-odd years, celebrated by having lunch together.

This year, Kate kept the appointment, but for the first time the reason for the rendezvous slipped her mind and she forgot to buy her fellow Capricorns birthday gifts. She was mortified and distressed. 'I mucked up … I knew the birthday lunch was coming up but somehow or other I forgot I had to have presents. So I offered to pay for the meal, which was rather clever of me!'[24]

Gorry later tells me that it was at the Capricorns' birthday bash about three years before, in 2001, that she and Annette first realised something was horribly wrong. Kate was not herself.

'She couldn't read the menu, the bill or the credit card slip … she battled to put on her jacket. Those were the first things we noticed.'[25]

In the album, Justine and Nicola's birthdays are documented, as are family holidays. Botswana, Sabi Sabi, the Drakensberg, Namibia, France. The Jowells went on holiday every June and December. Kate initiated and meticulously planned the trips.

'I thought them up and then talked to your pa about them,' Kate tells Justine. 'Then I went ahead and organised them.'

In 1988, it was Zimbabwe's turn. Kate met with trade unionist Morgan Tsvangirai – she had an instinct he would have an impact on the country's future – and made a pilgrimage to Bulawayo Convent. Justine points to the photograph showing her and Nicola flanking their mother in the school courtyard. Kate's eyes play tricks on her. Alzheimer's has affected her vision. Her finger trails off the photograph to the blank space next to it as she asks, 'Is that me?' We correct her, placing her finger on her tiny but distinct image. She has no recollection of the place or the moment.

Yet her years at Bulawayo Convent had been happy and successful. She got her O Levels when she was fifteen. Her father urged her to go to university – but Kate had other plans. She was in love. 'I was completely influenced by my first boyfriend, who thought university was a waste of time. My father was disappointed, though I did get a very good job.'[26]

This was with the income tax department of the then federal government of Rhodesia and Nyasaland. Within a year, she was doing tax assessments. 'It was most useful,' Kate jokes. 'I found out what my father earned!'[27]

She stayed on for two years, even starting a BComm degree by correspondence through the University of South Africa (UNISA). By then, however, she'd lost interest in both the job and the boyfriend. University beckoned. Big brother Paul had already started at UCT, studying physics and mathematics, when Kate joined him in 1958.

It was then that she made 'the most far-reaching decision of her life'.[28] Recounting her choice years later to journalist Zelda Gordon-Fish for a profile in *Cosmopolitan*, Kate explained: 'It was Freshers' Week and we all had to enrol in our chosen courses. There was a long line of students, 90 per cent girls, queuing up for the Arts course. There was a long line of students, also predominantly girls, queuing up for Social Science. But there was a shorter line of students, mostly male, queuing up for the sciences. I was good at maths, so I thought, "Why not apply for maths?", which I did.'

It was, as Gordon-Fish puts it, a seminal choice, 'a considered decision that indicated she had opted to join the men's club'.

Kate stayed in Denneoord, a boarding house just off the Rondebosch Main Road. There she met Doris Hollander, a medical student and fellow Rhodesian, who lived in the room next door. Doris's name comes up often in Kate's conversations – she is an ever-present character from Kate's childhood.

'Doris was older than me, and I was her sidekick. Her father was a lawyer who worked with my father. She is still around, in England somewhere.'[29] Doris's version of their association differs markedly from Kate's. 'I hardly knew Kathy [as a child]. I only knew her when we were living in the same rooming house in 1958 when we were studying.'[30]

The girls both hailed from Bulawayo, but the only thing Doris knew about Kate's background was that 'her father's business partner knew my father'. They were not close, and led separate lives. Even then, according to Doris, Kate was 'very sweet, but private and self-contained'.

'When I knew her she was very attractive, very, very neat and tidy. She was plumpish,' Doris adds, 'a peaches-and-cream type … a gorgeous-looking girl, with a lovely smile and laugh.'

Then there was the porridge and the piano playing. 'She always had porridge for breakfast, and she played the piano for the church every Sunday.'

The pair used to call each other 'Miss Kathy' and 'Miss Doris'. Kate, ever the mimic, has on many occasions rendered her version, hooting with laughter. Doris explains that they were fondly taking the mickey out of the Rhodesian domestic workers, who used to call the children of their white employers 'Miss This and Miss That'. They also shared a joke about Kate's Whitley Bay roots, the fact that the tiny village was in the sticks.

Since that time, they have kept up a communication of sorts. In 2001, when Doris, a psychiatrist who lives in England, eventually visited Whitley Bay, she emailed Kate. 'I finally went to Whitley Bay! Can you imagine! It was great. Much bigger than I expected. We had very good fish and chips. Nowadays it takes about thirty minutes by metro from Newcastle to get there. Best wishes, Doris.'

Kate herself contacted Doris in London, just before she retired. 'She was thin and gaunt, and seemed depressed,' Doris notes. Then she adds something others will tell me too. 'She's done most brilliantly, flying the flag for women and all that, but I didn't really get to know her at all.'

In 1960, Kathleen Bowman graduated with a BSc in Applied Mathematics. The year was a turning point, not only in her life, but also in South African history. For it was in 1960 that British prime minister Harold Macmillan made his famous 'Wind of Change' speech in Parliament in Cape Town, warning his South African counterpart, Hendrik Verwoerd, of the international shift towards decolonisation that would radically alter politics in Africa.

Verwoerd ignored the warning, of course, and a tumultuous time ensued – the Sharpeville shootings, the declaration of a state of emergency, and the banning of the African National Congress and the Pan Africanist Congress. Kate was convinced that the country 'had five years to go before it burst into flames'.[31] She went on to reflect, however: 'I realise now that I have suspect forecasting ability, but I always felt very temporary.'

So she left for London, for good. Or so she thought. 'Leaving South Africa for London was another major decision in my life. It broadened me, gave me new skills and good exposure. It got me out of Bulawayo – otherwise I might still be festering there today, who knows?'[32]

part two

JOURNEY
AWAY

4

London

(1961–63)

IN THE TWENTIETH century, every decade had its favourite city. In the sixties, that city was London, *TIME* magazine declared in April 1966.[33] It was a heady, vibrant time. London was, as Paul Bowman aptly puts it, 'a fun place'.[34]

After graduating from UCT in 1959 with a BSc, Paul changed his mind about doing postgraduate studies at Rhodesia's Salisbury University.[35] Instead, he asked his father if he could 'take off for England'. George Bowman was thrilled. 'My father realised then that Rhodesia had no future.'[36]

London, in stark contrast to most African cities, was humming. Although Paul didn't settle in the city – he lived and worked in Swansea, Wales, for a big company called Minnesota Mining – his move abroad prompted Kate to follow suit after completing her degree in 1960.

She arrived in 1961. London was a crucible of creativity. It was teeming with artists, models, pop stars, photographers, fashion designers and hairdressers, all dedicated and determined to create the decade's new look.[37] The Swinging Sixties had begun. 'Skirts got shorter, hair got longer ... and for the first time in the twentieth century, pop music became a driving force in society.'[38]

Enter the Fab Four: John Lennon, Paul McCartney, George Harrison and Ringo Starr – The Beatles – burst onto the London music scene in 1962 with their hit single 'Love Me Do'. They were so popular that, by

1963, 'Beatlemania' had spread to the rest of Europe and the United States. They recorded their songs at Abbey Road Studios in St John's Wood, which is where Kate, then Kathy Bowman, lived during her three-year stay in the British capital.[39]

Kate loved London life. She had just come of age, and she lived in a tiny bachelor flat that overlooked the hallowed Lord's cricket ground. 'She was a typical young woman,' Paul recalls. 'She was very confident, with a great sense of humour. Her humour has always been one of her most fabulous attributes.'[40]

Drawn to the world of financial journalism, she started working at a relatively obscure publication, *The Gold Mining Weekly*. Her impression today is that she worked on the paper 'for a very long time'. She was soon to move on, though, to the *Sunday Times* financial pages.[41]

More than forty years later, she remembers little, if anything, of this extraordinary time.

'I decided to work in England, so I went by boat, and I worked on a gold-mining newspaper,' she says eagerly. Then she loses the thread of her story. 'I had worked in a tax office in Zimbabwe, where they did books and things. A Greek girl worked in the media office with me. We all had lots of fun. There are other strands coming through … it's like a jigsaw puzzle that I have to piece together.'[42]

Kate did, indeed, have a Greek colleague, a warm, witty young woman whose overprotective mother called her every day to check on her comings and goings. The phone call was a standing joke between the two colleagues. But Kate's memory is letting her down, as the young women had, in fact, worked together at the Rhodesian tax department, not in a London media office.

Memory loss, or forgetfulness, is usually the first sign of Alzheimer's disease.[43] It is the single most common reason people seek medical help, according to doctors William Molloy and Paul Caldwell, authors of *Alzheimer's Disease*. They explain that 'a significant loss of the ability to remember is an essential factor in the diagnosis, so much so that the disease cannot be diagnosed unless it is present. You simply cannot have Alzheimer's disease and at the same time have normal memory.'

Kate's daughters Justine and Nicola, now grown women themselves, both trace the height of their mother's forgetfulness – before her progressive dementia was diagnosed in 1999 – to the mid-1990s. However, episodes of forgetfulness seem to have dogged Kate throughout the girls' childhood.

'In my mind,' Nicola recalls, 'Ma has always been forgetful, but she's always been so busy that I thought she was entitled to forget things.'[44]

However, in 1995, the year Nicola matriculated, she noticed that Kate, then fifty-five, was 'very absent-minded'.

Justine remembers that 'Ma', as the girls fondly call Kate, often forgot to fetch them from St Cyprian's – the private girls' school in Oranjezicht they attended from start to finish. 'A driver from my dad's work usually picked us up from school, but if we had something on, Ma would fetch us. Often, we'd wait and wait, until we realised, "Oh no, she's forgotten us again!" We'd have a good laugh, and we'd phone her.'[45]

At first Kate attributed her absent-mindedness to menopause. At the Business School, she began to feel less and less organised and unable to function with her usual efficiency. And when Justine was studying towards her BA degree in English and Politics at UCT from 1994 to 1996, she noticed that her mother was 'getting ditsier and ditsier'.[46]

'I remember feeling terribly frustrated because she seemed so slow. She would take ages to do things: if she had to pay for something, finding her credit card, signing the slip. It was a gradual decline. Basically, she just wasn't as sharp as she'd always been.'

But it was only once Justine had graduated and gone abroad that she realised the extent of Kate's problem.

'She came to visit me in London in 1997, and I remember being struck by the same thing. If we were in a shop, she always seemed to be in the way. I tried to put it down to her simply being distracted, and I thought that if she focused on the here and now she'd be okay and everything would be fine.'

But it was not the case. Kate's forgetfulness simply got worse and worse. It was a terribly traumatic time for her. For, as doctors Molloy and Caldwell point out, our sense of self, our identity, depends to a large degree on our ability to remember. 'We are all defined by our own specific collections of personal and distinctive experiences, encounters and achievements. These characterize us, delineate us, and all depend on our ability to recall the past at will. Our occupations, hobbies, interests, our learning and our relationships with others (even those we love) build layer on layer on what has gone before. Being unable to remember is a threat to our very being as thinking creatures.'[47]

If you can imagine a world where you can't trust your memory, where you can't recall the details of your life, you can begin to understand the fate of someone in the grip of Alzheimer's, a hugely complex, mystifying and terrifying disease that traps sufferers 'forever in the present, without any recourse to the past for understanding or comfort'.[48]

When I first met Kate Jowell, in the summer of 2002, she had already lived for four years with the knowledge that her brain was dying; that she was, for all intents and purposes, losing her mind. Her illness had already taken its toll, and Kate battled to make sense of its effects and consequences. At our first interview, shortly afterwards, she told me, 'What I understand about Alzheimer's – and this is the only thing I understand about Alzheimer's – is that I've got plaque on the brain.'[49]

This simple explanation is quite right, if selective. Alzheimer's disease is an affliction of the brain, and all its signs and symptoms are caused by damage to cells within the brain. 'The disease impairs the function of these cells at microscopic level, causing the deterioration in mental ability and behaviour that we observe on a day-to-day basis.'[50]

The 'markers' for Alzheimer's disease are the plaques and destructive fibres called 'neurofibrillary tangles' that accumulate in the brain and slowly but surely kill the brain's neurons, the nerve cells of which it is largely composed.[51] These 'neurofibrillary tangles' were first identified by a brilliant young German neurologist, Alois Alzheimer, in Frankfurt in 1905.

Four years prior to his ground-breaking discovery, Dr Alzheimer, a portly medical officer at a Frankfurt am Main mental asylum, encountered the patient who would become the first case study of the disease that would carry his name. We know the woman only as 'Auguste D'. This German housewife, who had an even, trusting temperament, had had a perfectly healthy, happy life until things began to change.

The first sign that something was amiss was her sudden fits of jealousy. Out of the blue, she grew suspicious of her husband and accused him of being unfaithful to her. Angry outbursts ensued. Then her memory began to fail her, and this led to more violent confrontations with her family. Her bewildered husband also began to find things in the oddest places – her hairbrush in the oven, his pipe in the laundry basket.

Then, her daily errand round became impossible. Auguste D could not find her way home. The situation deteriorated. She became confused and disorientated within the confines of her own apartment – she couldn't remember where the bathroom was, and forgot the names of simple household objects. She was no longer able to cook, or set the table. She also slept fitfully, and often woke up at night screaming. Finally, unable to cope, her desperate husband took her to the mental asylum, where Alois Alzheimer was the admitting neurologist.

Dr Alzheimer didn't recognise her condition, but it was clear that Auguste D had a progressive mental disease, and this doctor–patient encounter produced the first detailed description of a dementia that had not been officially recognised before; one that affected the middle-aged and those in their prime, like Kate Jowell.

Auguste D stayed in the asylum for four cruel, horrible years. Eventually, she failed to recognise not only herself, but also her husband and her family – and even Dr Alzheimer. The physician observed her decline, and it was only several days after she died, 'completely unaware of her surroundings ... bedridden ... incontinent, her legs drawn up and her arms curled across her chest ... a frail shell of the woman she had once been', that he could properly investigate the disease that had ravaged her.[52]

The patient's brain was removed from her skull and stained so that various cell types could be identified. The first thing the neurologist noticed was that the brain was lighter than usual, and that many of the expected brain cells were not visible: the neurons – responsible for all neurological thinking and activity – had disappeared. Also, many of the remaining neurons were not normal: 'In their cell bodies they had strange, threadlike, spindle-shaped objects that were very prominent.' In some cells the fibres were matted and thick, and appeared to be choking the neurons.

Dr Alzheimer called these filaments 'fibrils' (small fibres), labelling them 'neurofibrillary tangles', and their presence throughout the brain's outer layer – the cerebral cortex – is a diagnostic, microscopic sign of Alzheimer's disease. Auguste D's brain not only had 'neurofibrillary tangles' in abundance, but there were also prominent, viscous-looking blobs that Dr Alzheimer called 'plaques'. They had been identified before as senile plaques found in the brains of very old people.

'These three pathological changes in the brain – the loss of brain cells, the mats of destructive "neurofibrillary tangles" and the senile plaques – were Alzheimer's chief findings after he examined Auguste's brain,' note Molloy and Caldwell. 'A century later, they remain the basis for microscopic diagnosis of the disease.'[53]

As in the case of Auguste D, Alzheimer's disease struck Kate Jowell in the prime of her life. And so, if you ask her about her time in London in the psychedelic sixties, she cannot recall the sights, the sounds, the scenes of that highly memorable time. She has to rely on her family to do this for her. Paul Bowman says that, while she worked hard and worked well in London, she found the newspaper world 'very tough'.

'I don't think she enjoyed it that much,' he says.[54] He saw Kate as often as he could, travelling by car to London from Swansea to keep an eye on his younger sister.

Both siblings were mobile thanks to the generosity – and success – of George Bowman.

'We both got cars from Dad when we turned twenty-one,' Paul remembers. 'Kate turned twenty-one in London, and she got a red

Triumph Herald, which at the time was quite a car to drive. Needless to say, she loved it.'[55]

After three and a half years in England, Paul decided to return to Cape Town. But Kate stayed on for another year before she – and her Triumph Herald – came back in 1964. For the second time in her young life, she left England for Africa. This time, though, it would be for good.

5

Fair Lady

(1964–66)

'IT'S A GIRL! Born this month and pretty as a picture.' *Fair Lady*, South Africa's first English-language women's magazine, announced itself to the world on 6 March 1965. The cover line promised 'fashion and fiction, news and views, beauty and baby care, needlework and knitting, good cooking, good advice, sugar and spice and all things nice'. A pretty poppet, Leigh Crystal, all of three years old, graced the cover. Clad only in lacy bloomers and a string of pearls, she gingerly – and somewhat provocatively – sniffed at a posy of flowers.

A new era in magazine publishing had begun. Like its founding editor, Jane Raphaely, *Fair Lady* – as the title appeared back then – was revolutionary. Jane was a young, English-born go-getter who had just retired from running a PR agency for Bernstein Wilson when 'a bunch of Afrikaner gentlemen' at Nasionale Pers asked her to start a new magazine.[56]

'*Fair Lady* just happened to me,' Jane remembers. 'I was astonished to be offered the chance of starting an English-language women's magazine in a country I hardly knew.'[57]

Jane – today the CEO of her own company, Associated Magazines,[58] and the doyenne of South African women's magazine publishing – hand-picked a small, select team to get the magazine going. Her right-hand woman was Kathy Bowman.

Kate had returned to Cape Town from London by mail ship the year before, and she soon got a position at her alma mater, the University of Cape Town, tutoring students in the Applied Mathematics department.

Cape Town, however beautiful, must have seemed like a sleepy hollow after London. Still, it was a startling, eventful time characterised by political unease and tension in southern Africa. In Kate's native Southern Rhodesia, newly elected premier Ian Smith was threatening to declare unilateral independence (UDI). In South Africa, black activist Nelson Mandela – who was then serving a five-year prison sentence for incitement and leaving the country without a passport – and his fellow Rivonia trialists (including Walter Sisulu and Govan Mbeki), had been sentenced to life imprisonment. At the time, Mandela was commander-in-chief of the African National Congress's armed wing, Umkhonto we Sizwe.[59]

In what were decidedly interesting times, Kate soon got into the swing of Cape Town life. And, in one of the paradoxes of South African history, while black political movements fought for change, the lives of many whites flourished as never before. This was especially true of the young, gifted woman recently returned from London. Kate befriended an eccentric and talented journalist, Gorry Gordon Bagnall, and was soon living with Gorry and three other young women – Sue MacGregor, Sally Williams and Joy Forwell – in a charming, somewhat rundown Victorian house at 1 Kildare Road in the southern suburb of Claremont.

They were an intriguing bunch, destined for interesting lives. Gorry would marry the equally eccentric, flamboyant photographer Desmond Bowes Taylor and become a pioneering Cape Town newspaper journalist; Sue would become a legendary BBC radio personality, highly respected for her award-winning broadcast journalism in Britain; Sally would marry David, elder son of politician Sir De Villiers Graaff, the respected leader of the United Party and scion of one of the Cape's best-known families.

Sue MacGregor recalls with palpable nostalgia the house and its residents in her autobiography, *Woman of Today*. 'Number One Kildare Road,' she writes, 'had a sheltered patio at the back with an old fig tree. Three of the five of us had been at school together, so had no objection to sharing a small kitchen and one bathroom. I ran a taxi service into town each morning for as many as could squeeze into my Hillman Imp. We entertained regularly and quite a number of boyfriends were in evidence, though "staying over" was usually confined to Saturday nights. The sun warmed the house and made it seem a benign old place; we acquired a tabby cat called Wolsey who lazed about on the patio.'[60]

Sue remembers Claremont as a pleasant place to live. Parts of the suburb were still multiracial, and coloured families, some of them from the Cape Malay community, lived in 'little pockets of houses' beside their white neighbours. The Main Road mosque, and the muezzin's morning call from the tip of its tiny minaret, left a lasting impression on Sue. 'This call was, unusually, played on an old gramophone record; you could hear a tiny repetitive click behind it each time the faithful were summoned. From the Vineyard Fruit Supply in Protea Road opposite the house, you could buy grapes, avocado pears, melons, mielies – South African corn – and peaches.'

The population of the Claremont house waxed and waned as residents came and went. Gorry soon left to marry Desmond, 'as different from the average white South African male as it is possible to be: a firm royalist who wore a waistcoat, bow tie and watch chain, and a very skilful cook'. Sue's only reference to Kathy Bowman is that she was 'one of the early residents, a journalist from Rhodesia' – and that she was friendly with 'a quiet young lawyer called Albie Sachs'.[61]

Expanding on her published account of that time, Sue is unable to recall Kathy Bowman in any great detail. The two young women did not become firm friends, even though both were British expatriates who had migrated to Africa before they were ten years old.

Kathy, Sue recalls, was 'bespectacled, [with] short dark hair, very clever, funny, and much more "grown up" than the rest of us. I think for that reason she very quickly moved out of Number One Kildare Road, and I didn't see much of her after that.'[62]

Sue was working at the South African Broadcasting Corporation (SABC) at the time, running the afternoon magazine programme *Woman's World.* Three years later, in 1967, she would leave South Africa to join the BBC in London as a radio reporter, beginning an enduring professional association that earned her the accolade from *The Times*, 'Simply the best female presenter radio has produced' as, thirty years later, her career drew to a close.[63]

At the Claremont commune back in the 1960s, Kathy tended to keep to herself. 'I think she found some of us rather "irresponsible"! She was a fairly serious person,' Sue notes.[64]

Jenny le Roux, now the owner of Habits clothing boutique in Claremont, Cape Town, was not a resident, but 'an honorary member' of the house, as she was married. She confirms that the 'girls were as naughty as hell', and that Kathy usually tried to restore some sort of order.[65]

Today, Kate Jowell grins enigmatically when I ask her whether or not she disapproved of the frivolity and high jinks of 'the Kildare mob', as she calls them.

'Probably,' is all she will say. I can't pick up whether she's being characteristically discreet or whether the memory has been deleted, like so many others. She remains silent and I back off, not wanting to increase her distress at, once again, being unable to expand on a story, to recover her past.

To Sally Graaff, Kathy Bowman appeared ambitious, efficient, 'a together sort of person, and with that goes the success she made of her career. But she was almost old before her years.' Sally wryly admits that the house was 'slightly chaotic', something Kathy didn't like. 'She was very organised, and she certainly had a mind for detail. If you borrowed a spoonful of coffee from her, she'd be sure to ask for it back!'[66]

Like Sue MacGregor, Sally found Kathy aloof and 'not really my type'. Apart from being distant, Sue says, Kathy was also 'very discreet – unlike the rest of us! She did not approve of all the cars parked outside the house on Sunday mornings.'

At the time, Kathy's housemates assumed that she was romantically involved with Albie Sachs, but they were not entirely sure.[67] For even though Kathy Bowman shared her living space with a bunch of lively, interesting and stylish women, she preferred not to confide in them, and kept the intimate details of her life to herself. This urge for privacy and discretion at all costs soon became a character trait that would, in the future, alienate and intimidate many of her peers.

~

Albie Sachs is a man of rare and inspiring conviction. This legendary anti-apartheid activist, today a Constitutional Court judge, first met Kathy Bowman in 1964. She was teaching at UCT at the time, and he was a serious young Cape Town advocate at the Cape Bar.

When I approach him, Albie requests that, instead of an interview, we tape-record his recollections of their friendship. He warns that his portrait will be warm and intimate, and that he wishes to speak without interruption.

His face, though scarred by the car bomb that blew off his right arm and nearly ended his life in 1988 while he was living and teaching in Mozambique, is kindly and worn. His mind, however, is sharp. He sits at a wooden table in the open-plan lounge/dining-room area of his compact Clifton bungalow and begins to speak, without notes, but with much feeling, sometimes closing his eyes in concentration.

'Kathy stood out as someone different,' he says. 'It was not just the obvious things – the unfamiliar accent or the voice – it was the way she moved, the space she occupied. There was a spirit of independence about her. In those days, there were not many women lecturing at UCT, particularly in the fields of what I might call science. And she didn't dress to please men; she didn't make up her face to please men. She had a strong, independent way about her: not forceful, but determined; not aggressive, but assured. It was … just different.'[68]

Sachs explains that he was not unaccustomed to independent women. He had grown up in an activist, anti-racist, pro-worker Cape Town household. His father had been secretary of the Garment Workers' Union, and Albie had met many spirited, independent women – from trade unionists to 'struggle' comrades. 'Kathy had that same independence and spirit,' he says, but her sure sense of self, her singular vitality, was not part and parcel of a political movement, but simply 'of herself'.

Her willingness to engage with life left a lasting impression on Albie, one that he is able to recall, with vivid fluency, nearly forty years later. His ability to pinpoint the very essence of who she was – or was not – is remarkable. The Kathy Bowman Albie Sachs knew and loved was not someone who simply 'went along with things, snatching at small crumbs of satisfaction'. The goldfish idling in his patio pond suggest to him the metaphor that best delineates Kathy's truer nature. 'I watch the goldfish as they come up to nibble flakes of food. Some people go through life like that, immersed in a comfortable but not very exciting zone. They open their mouths momentarily to snatch at life. That wasn't Kathy. She engaged with life.'

The memory of how their friendship developed and matured, how they started going out and doing things together, eludes him, though he recalls that they had a close, provocative relationship.

'She was aware that I was deeply involved in the political struggle. I think she respected it as a fact. It was something that excluded her, in the sense that most of the work was underground, clandestine. It was a life that I had of intense and total significance to myself that she never intruded upon or wished to penetrate or sought to be included in. It was just part of me. Maybe she wasn't even fully aware of how much of my time and my thinking was devoted to the struggle. I had to hide it. So, I'm sure she would tease me' (he interrupts himself, confessing that he might merely be 'reconstructing this'), 'but I'm sure she would tease me for being monolithic in my preoccupations, tunnel-visioned, willing to expend my passion on an abstract cause and the suffering of others, rather than on myself and the intimacy of a personal relationship.

'I would "tease" her ... though "tease" isn't quite the right word ... I would throw out these little affectionate provocations about her correctness in the English style, little bits of manners, a kind of tight, correct way of seeing things and imagining oneself.'

But Sachs was curious about Kathy, about who she was, probably because he couldn't place her.

She didn't fit easily into any mould, he observes. 'If she'd been a third-generation Rhodesian farmer's child, she would have conformed to the

Doris Lessing kind of stereotype/non-stereotype. But she didn't. She wasn't a southern African lady. I gathered that her dad had been an artisan – I don't know if he was a fitter and turner or an engineer – a member of the skilled English working class who'd come to then Rhodesia and who'd been quite successful in business. The theme of what is now called "upward mobility" would have been quite strong – in class terms, but also in terms of imagination.

'Kathy wasn't stuck in an English industrial working-class worldview, having migrated to a new country, a new continent, and then being part of a family who had material success and a degree of comfort without being, I would call it, stricken by the mores of white upper-middle class southern African ladyship.'

The relationship was a very happy, comfortable one. It was also something of a haven, certainly for Sachs, who felt very secure with Kathy. She seemed isolated, and had a limited history in Cape Town.

'In that sense she was unencumbered, a free person. My relationship with her took place in a free and open space. It could develop its own spontaneous momentum. She gave me a great sense of security. I felt I could trust her, not only in the sense of never betraying me to the security police – that never arose because I don't recall sharing any secrets with her or asking her to hide documents or provide a safe house for me or anything like that. I mean emotional trust. There was something steady and decent and honourable about her that I liked very much.'

Nineteen sixty-four was but one of the many 'exceptionally intense' moments in Albie Sachs's remarkable life. He was twenty-nine years old at the time.

'The security police were closing in,' he says. 'They were cracking down – arresting people, torturing and killing people in detention.'

Some of his clients had been tortured to death. And he knew many people who had been detained in solitary confinement for long periods. He lived with the constant fear and tension of being locked up himself. Understandably, his trusting relationship with Kathy was especially important to him. She knew he was in danger, but she didn't abandon him. Her emotional strength, her physical affection, the way she lived her life, provided a glow to his life.

~

Kate Jowell clearly remembers the Albie Sachs of the 1960s.

'I was very taken with him, he is a very soft sort of man,' she confides.

It is interesting that she is able to relive intimate moments with Sachs all these years later, despite the progress of her disease.

'He was an advocate at the time,' she continues. 'We had a friendship, and then it became a bit more than that …' Her voice trails off, as it sometimes does when she battles from within the confines of her now limited world to engage with and articulate the details of her once complex life.[69]

We are at Carlucci's, our familiar haunt. In a marked way, Alzheimer's disease is slowly tightening its grip. Sometimes, as Kate starts to speak, words that bear no relation to each other tumble from her mouth. Exasperated and bewildered, she will say, with painful resignation, 'I'm not making myself clear. Let's just leave it.'

It is all deeply distressing – for Kate, and for those close to her. But there are still good days, like today, when she is warm and responsive – even though her memory fails her at times. She is visibly intrigued, and moved, when I tell her of Albie Sachs's tribute to her. But she is shocked to learn of the horrific car-bomb attack during his exile in Mozambique in 1988, while he was living and working in Maputo. Sachs lost not only his right arm, but also the sight in one eye. His legs were badly damaged, and his hearing was partly impaired. 'I don't remember that at all,' Kate says, clearly shaken by news that had made international headlines at the time.

We move on, and she is delighted to hear of his recollections of the quaint Rosebank cottage she had made her own when she took her leave of 'the Kildare mob'. Albie says Kathy was 'quite excited' when she found 20 Ayres Road. He, in turn, found the place 'quite startling' in more ways than one.[70]

'It was a little cottage, and in those days young progressive profession-als aspired to a nice, bright flat in a modern building. It seemed strange to me that a young, progressive person should want to go into an old cottage. But, again, Kathy was a precursor in that sense. Today, young progressive people favour living in cottages and look on bright, modern flats with disdain.'

Also, Sachs was uneasy about the fact that people classified as coloured who had lived in Rosebank had been evicted from the area, and from their homes, under the Group Areas Act.

'The properties had now been developed as desirable little homes and it hurt me, and I felt this unease and discomfort at being happy in Kathy's company, and enjoying her delight in a place that had become available through dispossession.'

Interestingly enough, he didn't raise his concerns with Kathy. I won-der what compelled him to remain silent, but I am all too aware of his request that I ask no questions.

The cottage was very much her space, he continues. She put a lot of thought into its furbishing and furnishing. Sachs can no longer visualise the place, but he remembers enjoying the fact that she'd chosen the cottage, and that she had a vision of how she wanted it to look.

And it was not on Albie Sachs alone that the cottage made an impact. Veteran South African journalist Cathy Knox also remembers it as a unique place. Cathy had first met her namesake at the *Fair Lady* offices. By late 1964, Kathy Bowman had left UCT for the glamorous, exciting environment of pioneering magazine journalism. It was, in many ways, a radical shift, from the precision of the world of mathematics to the somewhat wayward world of magazines. But, having cut her teeth on British business newspapers, she would have felt confident and at home returning to journalism, albeit the world of women's magazines. Also, she had met, and befriended, Jane Raphaely, who, knowing Kathy's background in financial journalism, offered her a sought-after, enviable position as the new magazine's assistant editor.

Kathy was clearly intrigued and, like so many others, found it hard to say no to Jane. In any case, this was the opportunity of a lifetime.

Fair Lady was breaking new ground as South Africa's first English-language women's magazine, and Jane Raphaely became the first female editor of a South African women's magazine. The Afrikaans women's magazines at that time were all edited by men – a rather peculiar tradition that would continue for at least twenty years.

Jane's appointment was questioned in some business circles. 'The *Financial Mail* was startled and wrote a knocking piece which suggested that Nasionale was *deurmekaar* (confused). What would they have said if they'd realised that Hubert Coetzee and his colleagues knew I was pregnant when they offered me the job and were aware that the magazine and the baby were due at the same time?' Jane muses.[71]

Cathy Knox joined the magazine as a junior staffer in 1966. She stayed in a Rosebank flat a stone's throw from Kathy Bowman's cottage. For a long time, Kathy gave her a lift to work.

Cathy used to go across to the cottage every morning. She'd find Kathy sitting at the table – on which there was always a vase with fresh flowers – having her breakfast. 'She was very much the lady, but in a friendly, relaxed way. Her cottage was gorgeous. It was filled with scraped-down oak and Oregon pine furniture with rugs scattered on the wooden floors.'[72]

Kathy had excellent taste, and 'she had all the goodies': Marimekko bowls in just the right colours, imported Casa Pupo pieces. 'She was always in tune with the 1960s style, but she was not experimental. She was not all over the place like a lot of us were in those days.'

Cathy Knox soon became the magazine's teenage editor, and reported directly to Kathy Bowman, her older mentor. 'She was quite scary in a way – I knew I could not pull a fast one on her. My first impression of her was that she seemed a lot older than I was, even though I was nineteen and she was twenty-six at the time.'

Cathy found her boss to be an excellent teacher, who always made time to talk to her and tell her things. 'She checked everything I did, and she didn't give me a chance to dig a hole and fall into it ... she was very kind, very fair.'[73]

At the time, Kathy Bowman's task encompassed more than overseeing

Cathy Knox's work. She was also in charge of *Fair Lady*'s fashion, food and decor (called 'homemaking' at the time) departments. In fact, one of the first pieces she set up and wrote, 'Home on a Shoestring', advised newlyweds Jenny le Roux and her husband, Jeffrey, on how to furnish their mews flat for just R150. In her crisp style, Kathy wrote:

> *Jennifer and Jeffrey set up house on the proverbial shoestring. Their first home is a one-room mews flat in Cape Town's Newlands, one of a row, newly converted from old labourer's cottages. 'We wanted to rent a furnished flat to start with, as our honeymoon and the boat trip from England ate up most of our capital,' said Jenny, 'but when we saw this we just had to take it. But how on earth can we make it liveable on our minute income and non-existent savings?' Well, we thought it was possible, if not for nothing, at least on the comparatively small budget of R150. Fair Lady invested the money and hours of good advice, and Jennifer invested all her free time and enthusiasm in the project. Eventually, as the pictures show, Jennifer got her furnished flat, and we proved our point.*

The team were 'all rather sorry' when the assignment came to an end, 'but we hope that the next young couple who come to *Fair Lady*'s Homemaking department will tell us that money is no object, and exercise our talents in a different direction!'[74]

Today, Jenny le Roux clearly remembers the story as she sits in her office at Habits (which, interestingly, is just down the road from the Kildare Road commune). She reveals that she, too, was terrified of Kathy.

'I was terribly disorganised at the time, and I had to run around looking for furniture and stuff. Every time Kathy came round she'd find me asleep. She was so organised, *and* she was bossy!' Jenny also admits, with characteristic candour, that a reason for her being intimidated by a 'strict and stern' Kathy was that she was 'fresh out of tutoring maths at UCT'.[75]

As I reread the magazine article, I imagine a prim and proper Kathy Bowman concluding it:

We wanted to show that with colour co-ordination, careful allocation of space and money, and consideration of the needs of the people who have to live in the home they make, a home can be furnished on a shoestring and still look as welcoming and well thought out as if our newlyweds had been millionaires.

In my interview with her, Jenny carefully considers Kathy Bowman's talents, and goes on to label her as very ambitious, though she quickly adds that people had great respect for her. It comes as no surprise therefore that Jane Raphaely credits Kathy Bowman with being 'an excellent assistant editor'.[76]

At the time, *Fair Lady* operated from the Nasionale Tydskrifte headquarters in Keerom Street, Cape Town – the magazine division of Afrikaans media giant Nasionale Pers. Eileen Snowball, one of the first *Fair Lady* staffers, describes the building that housed the group's magazines and newspapers: 'The magazines were all on one level, along with the photographic department. We worked in a warren of partitioned offices with khaki linoleum floors, no air conditioning and little space.'[77]

Fair Lady had a small staff of six – including Kathy Bowman – and shared its art department with *Sarie*, one of Nasionale's first Afrikaans magazines for women. The new magazine 'hit the 100 000-copy mark very quickly in that first year'.[78] It was 'quite different from anything we had in South Africa at the time', and soon earned roomier, more comfortable space in the Keerom Street offices. As Eileen – who worked in the art department first of *Sarie* and then of *Fair Lady* – recalls, 'Rumour had it that the board of directors at Nasionale Pers weren't that fluent in English, and whenever Jane asked for something, confused by her English accent, they just said "Yes".' The team ended up working in what was then the lap of luxury – a spacious office, complete with air conditioning and carpets.

It was a glamorous milieu. Keerom Street, close to the Cape Town High Court, had a cosmopolitan feel, thanks, in part, to what Eileen refers to as a bunch of 'Swiss-Italian boys'. *Fair Lady* had 'imported' them to train experts in the photographic field who were not au fait with colour photography and black-and-white retouching – at the time the latest photographic technology.

'Most of them were very handsome, and the street was also full of their sports cars – all of which added a touch of exotic glamour to the area. Truworths had its head office nearby and its young buyers used to be in and out wearing the latest fashions, which they'd bought overseas. It was heady stuff for a young girl!'[79]

But, Eileen admits, for all the glamour and the applause, it was hard work and 'sometimes a bit crazy'. For one, the editor 'seemed to be pregnant all the time for the first couple of years'. Indeed, Jane Raphaely had two of her four children – her second-eldest daughter Vanessa, followed fairly closely by youngest daughter Julia – in the early years of *Fair Lady*'s conception. Her youngest child, Paul, a *laatlammetjie* (late-come child), was born much later.

Kathy Bowman, who was very close to Jane at the time, was a stable presence on the magazine. Self-contained and extremely practical, she never became hysterical or overexcited under pressure. She had her finger on *Fair Lady*'s pulse.

'There was an air of peace and balance around her,' Cathy Knox says. 'She was very quiet, and her appearance was very soft. Her face was round, and her eyes were too. She was plumper then. I remember she had a pair of very good pearl earrings, which she wore with her Biba clothes. She didn't favour the loud, colourful clothes of Mary Quant. She was a Biba girl.'[80]

Biba, the brainchild of Polish designer Barbara Hulanicki, was the first London label to make street fashion hip and cool in the Swinging Sixties.[81] Kathy had probably bought her Biba collection while she was still living in the British capital. The clothes would have satisfied her yen to be stylish, but would also have appealed to her conservative, cautious nature. For not only did Hulanicki favour funereal colours – blacks and browns and dark, plummy purples – but her creations were also considerably cheaper than those of Mary Quant.

At the back of Cathy Knox's mind there was always the notion that her mentor, whom she found to be very bright, was merely working at a glossy women's magazine to hone her homemaking skills. Still single, she enjoyed a friendship with Jane's brother-in-law Johnny Raphaely, but he was not a serious suitor.

Today, Kate Jowell strains to remember it all, as she wistfully recalls having known Johnny Raphaely. 'I'm just trying to remember ... Johnny was a lovely man.'[82]

In the recording of his memoir of Kathy Bowman, Albie Sachs refers to the 1960s as being a time of 'personal liberation'. It gave individuals the 'capacity to enjoy sex, to have a full relationship ... not to satisfy the expectations of society, not in the framework of establishing a family and marriage and everything that went with that, but simply as an intense interpersonal encounter'.[83]

At the time, Kathy, an active correspondent, had written a letter to her mother, Kathleen, about the men in her life. Intriguingly, she revealed the contents of the letter to Albie Sachs: 'She told her mother that there were three men in her life at that stage – X, Y and Z. X had certain qualities, Y had others, but the most interesting one was Z – that was me.'

Was she subtly manipulating the situation, or was it indicative of a remarkable degree of emotional detachment? When I ask him, Sachs expresses uncertainty. 'I don't know if that was her way of getting our relationship on the agenda so that we could talk about it – or if it was part of her intellectually cool way of observing the world around us and ourselves.'

One of the strengths of the relationship was that there was 'no drama', and while it was loving, warm and affectionate, there was no 'deep sense of destiny and overwhelming commitment'. Sachs, who was consumed by his political activism, seems to have missed the signs that this relationship was not enough for Kathy Bowman. For she was after a sense of destiny, a firm commitment – something Albie was neither willing to nor capable of offering.

'I think, from my part,' he says, 'I couldn't have loved – to the point of total distraction – someone who didn't share the vision and the danger and the experience of underground work.' The struggle was his *raison d'être*. Kathy, on the other hand, 'wanted and required someone whose passion was expressed in a far more intimate and interpersonal way'. While for Sachs the personal and the political were indivisible, for Kathy – in his view – the personal was all.

Albie Sachs never pried into her personal life. He was part of it – 'but just a part. She had a life right outside me.'

~

Significantly, in her 'nice, interesting but orderly' office, Kathy Bowman had cut out from a classy British magazine and stuck on her pinboard a picture depicting the ultimate happy family.[84]

'It was from a breakfast-cereal ad,' Cathy Knox recalls, 'and it was beautifully styled and shot, with lovely light streaming in through the window.'

Kathy Bowman pinned it in a very prominent place – and she kept it there. Cathy Knox cannot recall whether or not Kathy ever told her of its meaning or importance to her. 'I may have surmised it, but it was clear that that was what she thought was an ideal family, a happy family. I got the strong impression that it represented something that she was seeking in her own life. I felt that she was definitely looking for a husband.'

Unbeknown to everyone – friends and family – Kathy had by then met the man who would, eventually, become her husband. Looking back, Albie Sachs recalls that Kathy suddenly left Cape Town for London, and 'there was a hint that something quite significant was stirring in her life. I had the sense that there was someone, a fellow, at the other end. At the time I thought, well, it's just another addition to X, Y and Z.'

As it turned out, Albie Sachs had misjudged the situation completely. Kathy Bowman was in great turmoil. She had finally met the love of her life.

6

Love and Marriage

(1966–70)

I N MANY RESPECTS, Neil Jowell was an extremely eligible prospect.
The eldest son of the legendary Joe Jowell, Namaqualand businessman and community giant, Neil was a UCT law graduate who'd worked
in the highly successful Jowell family business in Springbok for a few
years before leaving for New York to do an MBA at Columbia University.
A two-year working spell in London followed before he returned to
Cape Town.

Neil met Kathy Bowman sometime in 1966. 'I think the first time I
saw her was at a friend's New Year's Eve party,' Neil recalls. 'I can't quite
remember.'

The details of their encounter are blurred. And Kate, similarly, has
no real recollection of seeing Neil for the first time. But the attraction
between them was strong and instant. Neil was struck by her intelligence,
her ability to cut to the quick, to see things clearly and put them in perspective.

'She had such a clear mind, and a great sense of humour, which I liked.
And she obviously thought I was funny too, because, unlike everyone
else, she laughed at my jokes!'[85]

Their meeting, and subsequent love affair, would dramatically change
both their lives. Kathy Bowman had finally found the man of her dreams,
and a 'relationship with deep, intense passion that would be really mean-

ingful to her'.[86] Neil Jowell encountered a compelling, clever career woman who was ahead of her time, who captured his imagination, and also his heart. They fell in love, but there was one serious problem: Neil was married, with three small boys.

It must have been a terrifying yet exhilarating situation for Kathy Bowman. Caught up in a passionate affair with a dashing, clever and wealthy man, she no doubt baulked at the idea of intruding on his marriage, of taking him away from his wife, Bertha, and his sons, David, Paul and Michael. Confused and distressed, she nonetheless allowed Neil to pursue her, and they began a secret affair that would culminate in their marriage four years later.

The intervening years were difficult. On several occasions Kate has been at pains to explain to me that it was Neil who pursued her, Neil who was 'determined' that they would be together.[87]

But the untangling of his marriage took its toll, and for someone who lived her life in a meticulous, precise and principled way, she must have found the situation hard to bear. Yet, true to her discreet and private nature, she revealed nothing of her inner distress to the outside world. Not even Jane Raphaely, her close friend (and also her boss at *Fair Lady*), knew that she was involved with Neil, and that her life had been plunged into chaos.

'She didn't talk about it. I had no idea she was seeing Neil Jowell,' Jane recalls.[88]

After the relationship inevitably became public, Kathy was 'not really involved in most of the commotion', for she had escaped to London for three months to give Neil space and time to make up his mind about his future.[89] Neil recalls: 'After we got together, she said, "Look, let me go away for three months and you can make up your mind without any pressure." So she went away, to London.'

Albie Sachs remembers taking leave of Kathy, and sensing that she was disappointed at not being able to confide in him at a time she sorely needed his consolation and advice.

'I was not able to encompass the drama that she was going through, even though I was her confidant – not simply a passive, listening, platonic confidant, but an intimate, close, loving confidant,' he says with some regret. 'I should have given her more support.'[90] But the details of the relationship were 'shrouded'. 'There was no name, no context, no personality,' Albie explains. 'It only emerged afterwards that she'd become involved with Neil.'

Sachs remembers Kathy finding the situation complex and difficult. 'It was clear that Neil had intense feeling for her, and it was clear that his marriage had already come to an end.'

Still, Cape Town society judged the couple harshly, and perhaps inevitably Kathy, as the 'other woman', bore the brunt of this. One of Kathy's former house mates, a member of the Kildare mob, who had found her 'prissy and judgmental', says they were all surprised when they discovered she was involved with Neil Jowell: 'We never thought she would go off with someone else's husband.'[91]

Sachs can recall overhearing similarly hurtful, derogatory comments about the scruples and principles of the couple. He was tempted on more than one occasion to set the record straight.

'It cost me a lot to maintain the privacy of my friendship with Kathy, not to be able to say that she was in total turmoil, that she was intensely drawn to Neil, that she felt the power of his love, that she didn't initiate or provoke the situation at all, and she was unsure of what to do.'

Confiding to me in his Clifton bungalow, Albie Sachs says, with palpable sadness, that he failed her during this period. 'Instead of being a person to whom she could speak without fear of the information being abused in any way, the person who could give her courage and strength to do what was right – whatever that was – I just carried on in that kind of provocative, jokey-jokey way that had characterised our friendship.'

His apparently superficial naivety angered a tormented Kathy, even though she knew he was unaware of the problems, the huge challenge and the heartache that had beset her. She wrote him a 'very harsh' letter, which he took as a sign that their relationship had come to an end. 'It was very different from anything we'd ever said or done, a denunciation that I took as her way of saying that in order to move on with her life, it was necessary to sever our ties,' he says.

While her relationship with Sachs could not impede the strong, passionate bond she now had with Neil, Kathy still needed to choose one or the other, 'for her own internal, emotional clarification'. She lashed out at Sachs partly because it was traumatic for her to cut ties with him. She loved him, she recognised his exceptional qualities, she admired his dedication to the liberation struggle, she valued their friendship and the meaningful way they had connected, physically and intellectually. But she could not, or would not, let their relationship overlap or cloud her intense bond with Neil Jowell.

Sachs, on the other hand, believed it was quite possible for his friendship with Kathy to continue. He concedes that he is 'often naive about these things', assuming that friendships can 'carry on independently of context'.

In 1966 he went to London, and like many anti-apartheid activists at the time, into political exile. He is not clear about whether he met up with Kathy there, or whether he merely tried to contact her, and whether his efforts to communicate with her came before or after that sharp and angry letter. By then, he was already married to Stephanie Kemp, who had followed him to London. Even under these circumstances, he still assumed that he and Kathy could remain close friends.

'I'd assumed that the affectionate, confidential type of friendship – now without a physical dimension and far less intimate – could have continued beyond my marriage and beyond her new relationship.'

Again, he concedes, 'people are different in that respect', and it is possible that his assumption represented an unwitting insensitivity on his part.

Kathy rejected Albie Sachs, it appears, in a rather ruthless manner. Perhaps she had it in her to be cold and calculating at a time of inner turmoil. But from another perspective, she was simply being true to herself, allowing her instinct for simplicity and clarity to take hold. For if an already muddied situation were to become more clear-cut for her, Albie Sachs, whom she had loved perhaps more than she'd realised, could no longer be a part of her life.

In London, while she was waiting for Neil to make a decision, she underwent a telling metamorphosis. Not only did she change her first name from Kathy to the crisper Kate, but she also lost ten kilograms, extra weight that had dogged her for most of her life and earned her tags such as 'round', 'plump' and 'soft'. She emerged, like a butterfly from its chrysalis, stylish and confident, a young woman on the cusp of an exciting new life.

Jenny le Roux remembers Kate's striking transformation: 'She had been plump and became sylph-like, and adamant about the way she wanted to look. She suddenly changed into a very well-turned-out woman. We should have known there was a man in her life!'

But Jenny and the Kildare girls would never have guessed that the man was Neil Jowell. 'Kathy was such a private person; we didn't really know what kind of man she'd find attractive,' Jenny says.[92]

Many people assume that Neil was behind this radical reinvention, that he urged Kate to lose weight and to change her name. But while Neil's arrival in her life signalled a shift in the way she perceived and presented herself, he was merely the catalyst, not the cause. When I asked her why she had felt it necessary to change her name at the age of twenty-six, when she already had a clear identity as Kathy Bowman, she replied, 'I was christened Kathleen, which was my mother's name, but people always called me Kath or Kathy. Later on I became Kate because I wanted to distinguish myself from my mother, and I could do it by changing my name.'[93]

Kathleen Bowman senior was a striking woman. Kate got on with her, and loved her, but she was closer to her father – for she was the apple of George Bowman's eye. And when her love affair with Neil Jowell changed forever the sense she had of herself as a woman, she blossomed. Her choice of the succinct, strong 'Kate' above the softer derivative, 'Kath', is revealing. With the exception of her family, no one called her Kath or Kathy ever again.

Her metamorphosis complete, Kate Bowman returned to Cape Town. Soon afterwards, Neil Jowell moved into Kate's Rosebank cottage in Ayres Road.

~

He is a difficult man to place. As executive chairman of Trencor Ltd – the company started by his father, Joe Jowell, in 1929 (originally Jowells Garage & Transport) – Neil Jowell is powerful, successful and, in his wife's words, 'a very wealthy man'. But he does not seem to need to play the part. He is also not particularly interested in an outward show of wealth. His Foreshore office at Trencor is neither especially big nor grand. In fact, its overriding feature is its spectacular view of Table Mountain, offered by the wall-to-wall windows that rattle when the notorious Cape Doctor blows. From here, when he has a moment to spare, Neil takes in the impressive cityscape. From his desk, he can see as far as his Glencoe Road home high against the mountain, in Gardens.

Our first meeting, in January 2003, to discuss my writing a book on Kate's life and her illness, takes place here. A commanding, affable man, Neil speaks quickly, almost swallowing his words as they spill out of his mouth. He is not especially eloquent, though, when business or cycling – his other passion – is not on his mind. Often, his gaze is inscrutable and steady, and downright unnerving. Kate will later explain that he is shy.

But for all his apparent reticence, Neil Jowell is not afraid to show his feelings, which is perhaps unusual for a man of his generation and social stature. For when our conversation turns to Kate's debilitating and devastating disease and her prognosis, this imposing man is overcome with emotion and is forced to stop speaking.

Later when I meet with Neil, it's at Glencoe Road once his hectic working day has ended. We sit in the study he has shared with Kate for close on three decades. The room is a small, efficient personal space. The desks are placed diagonally opposite one another, complete with separate bookshelves. The shelves above Kate's desk are almost empty – since Alzheimer's has taken hold, she has rummaged indiscriminately through her things, often discarding books and files, ironically deleting her own history as her physical decline progresses.

Neil's shelves reveal his interests – there are Trencor annual reports, a copy of George Soros's *Open Society*, books on cycling, his Smuts Hall mug from his UCT days. A third, communal floor-to-ceiling bookshelf is crammed with an array of interesting titles: Kate's interest in and love of cooking is evident (there are many recipe books), as is her eclectic interest in literature: Margaret Drabble, Saul Bellow, Günter Grass, Paul Theroux, Iris Murdoch, JM Coetzee, Mike Nicol. And so on.

Before Alzheimer's laid claim to her abilities and interests, Kate Jowell was a formidable reader – of fiction as well as non-fiction. The wide range of reading matter attests to her insatiable intellectual appetite, her eagerness to engage with the world, to challenge her perceptions, to broaden her knowledge. There is also a clutter of photographs on the bookshelves, documenting the school years of Justine and Nicola, and of Neil's boys in the various stages of their lives.

Above Kate's desk are faded family portraits of her parents, of her brother, Paul, and of herself as a chubby little girl. When I visit Kate we often end up here, at her desk, where I comb her filing cabinets and bookshelves for clues to her life. Her once meticulously tidy and organised desk is now invariably in disarray, with papers and photographs strewn over its blond wood surface. She spends a lot of time sitting here – at the desk where she produced some of her most important papers – just sifting and sorting mindlessly, it seems, through her life, in a desperate attempt to make sense of it, to give it an order and a logic that are slowly but steadily seeping away.

Neil's personal memorabilia include various artistic offerings from his grandchildren, but there are no photographic clues to his own childhood. Scanning the shelves behind his desk, my eyes inevitably fall on a thick volume with a stone-coloured spine, *Joe Jowell of Namaqualand – The Story of a Modern-day Pioneer*; the biography of his charismatic father, written by Phyllis Jowell, wife of his brother Cecil.[94] That is the only clue the shelves yield.

The Jowell family history is fascinating. Neil himself is a fourth-generation South African Jowell, heir to the remarkable talent and wealth of a courageous Jewish immigrant family. As Phyllis Jowell's biography reveals, the forebears of Joe and Bessie Jowell (she was born Rebecca Berelowitz, though everyone called her Bessie) were immigrant Jews from Lithuania in Eastern Europe. The Jowells' original home town was Plungyan, the Berelowitz's Ponevesz. Sometime in the late 1800s, Joe's grandfather (and Neil's great-grandfather) Abraham made his way to the southern tip of Africa to seek new opportunities and a better life.

Abraham, a *smous* (hawker), sold goods to people scattered throughout the dry, desolate hinterland to the north of Cape Town. He arrived in Namaqualand in 1880, having left his three small children behind in Lithuania. He was thirty-seven. Abraham was concerned about the discriminatory Lithuanian practice of military conscription for Jewish boys – he had two sons, Herman and Isaac, and a daughter, Feige.

Determined to bring his boys to Africa, Abraham worked hard for ten years, trekking from farm to farm with his mule-drawn cart to ply his trade, before he could afford to send for Herman and Isaac. By then Herman was twenty-one. He joined his father, and together they crisscrossed Namaqualand. In 1898, Abraham Jowell died when his cart overturned while descending the steep Kamiesberg.

By now Herman was twenty-nine years old. He was naturalised in 1899 and followed his mother's family to Paarl. He eventually set up a trading store in the small settlement of Riebeek West, and his brother Isaac did the same, in neighbouring Riebeek Kasteel. Herman bought a property and married Dora Shapiro of Paarl, 'a capable, confident, beautiful woman'. The couple had five children: Abraham, who was called Abe after his grandfather, Joseph (Joe), Simon (Simie), Ida and Esme.

'Joe had bad eyesight as a result of a trachoma,' Phyllis writes in *Joe Jowell of Namaqualand*. By the time they got Joe to a doctor, when he was already two years old, he had lost most of the sight in his right eye and had limited vision in his left eye.[95]

But this disability was not to deter Joe Jowell. He grew up in Riebeek West but attended Paarl Gymnasium – today a highly regarded Afrikaans-medium boarding school – from the age of nine. There he learnt bookkeeping, and would often help his father with his accounts, cycling ten kilometres home from school.

Joe was hard-working, determined and ambitious, but he was not an exceptional student. When he matriculated in 1922 at the age of seventeen, he obtained a second-class pass. University beckoned, and he registered to study law at UCT. There he met Bessie Berelowitz, the woman who would become his wife.

Bessie had come to South Africa with her family in 1906. The youngest daughter of a rabbi, the Reverend Solomon Berelowitz, Bessie, like Kathy Bowman, was a woman ahead of her time. 'She did a Bachelor of Arts degree, majoring in Zoology, at a time when there were very few women at university,' Neil says. 'She was a remarkable person.'[96]

In 1924, the year Bessie graduated with her BA and a Secondary Teacher's Lower Certificate, Joe passed his Law Certificate exams. Two years later he was admitted as an attorney. But Joe's destiny did not lie in the legal profession: his eyes had weakened further during his years of studying, his finances were not good and he had begun to suffer from excruciating migraines. So, when he was offered a business partnership in a garage that had the GM franchise in the remote Namaqualand town of Springbok, he eagerly took the opportunity. The following year he married his Bessie in rural Calvinia, her home town. 'I had the good sense to marry her on her birthday, and that has saved me forty presents already,' Joe once revealed rather mischievously in an interview.[97]

After their honeymoon, the Jowells embarked on what would soon become their remarkable life in Springbok.

⌒

There were 2 000 people living in the town when Joe and Bessie set up home in Springbok. A thriving mining village before its copper mines were shut down in 1919, Springbok survived because of its location – it was in the centre of Namaqualand. Ten years later it had become the capital of the region, and the discovery of diamonds in 1927 reignited the town's commercial prospects.

Things went well for Joe and Bessie right from the start. Joe was in equal partnership with Jaap du Plessis in a company called JD du Plessis & Co. Car sales soared. But by 1930, Springbok was feeling the effects of the Great Depression, precipitated by the Wall Street crash of October 1929. The area was also experiencing one of the worst droughts of the century. Then, without warning, the South African Railways withdrew its motor service from the railhead at Bitterfontein to Springbok.

'Within a fortnight, panic reigned. Who else to turn to but the garage, no matter that they did not possess even a single truck?'[98] Jaap and Joe gamely rose to the challenge, building a vehicle – part car, part truck – which did the job, even though it was overloaded by three to four times its capacity.

'For the next three years Du Plessis and Jowell took turns at managing (during the day) and truck driving (during the night) – with a shower in between. Mrs Jowell, meanwhile, was receptionist, book-keeper and secretary and the partners now owned some 45 trucks.'[99]

Business was booming, and Joe didn't have a chance to 'plan the next step'. And he was soon an involved and influential member of the Springbok community. A music lover – he could play several instruments, the violin being his favourite – he was asked to join the town's first syncopated dance band.

Then, when he was twenty-eight – and while Bessie was pregnant with Neil – Joe became the youngest member of the Springbok Municipal Council. Four years later, in 1937, he was elected mayor, a position he would hold, with two interruptions, for more than twenty-five years.

Joe Jowell was not, however, a small-town mayor. The world was his oyster, and he soon became a national and international business figure. A tenacious and driven character, he believed that the only way to the top was by 'ordinary hard work'. And work hard he did. In the mid-1940s he bought out Jaap du Plessis and renamed the business Jowells Garage & Transport, buying not only vehicles on a large scale, but also his first aeroplane. His vision, coupled with his business success, had a phenomenal impact on the development of Springbok and of the entire Namaqualand region. For Joe, a Namaqualander through and through, was determined to put the town on the map.

Then, in 1947, Joe's health took a turn for the worse when he suffered the first of many blackouts. His doctors diagnosed complete heart block, aggravated by the onset of Stokes-Adams attacks – total blackouts brought on when the pulse rate drops to eighteen (an average pulse rate is between sixty and seventy). But, true to his independent, energetic nature, Joe ignored his doctor's orders to slow down. His only concession was never to go anywhere on his own, and Bessie loyally accompanied him everywhere, until Neil and Cecil took over from her.

In 1961, Joe became known as 'the flying mayor' when Jowells Garage & Transport started the Namakwaland Lugdiens, which in those days had two twin-engine aircraft. The company operated a passenger service between Cape Town and Springbok five days of the week, and one charter out of Springbok. Both Neil (who was a trained South African Air Force pilot) and Cecil flew the aircraft, and they often ferried Joe about on business trips.

By the mid-1960s, Jowells – which had a virtual monopoly on road transport in Namaqualand – had diversified into engineering and manufacturing, and became Transport & Engineering Investment Corporation Limited – Trencor. 'Our company has continued to progress solidly,' Joe Jowell stated in the 1966 company report.[100]

The acquisition of the Johannesburg-based Henred Trailer Engineering Company in 1967 was an especially important turning point for Jowells. And it was at this time that Joe's sons, Neil and Cecil, became a major force in the business. Neil Jowell was, at that point, living with his family in London, where he worked for United Transport; prior to that, he had worked for Esso Oil in New York for eighteen months. But he now decided to return home to head the Cape transport section of the family business. At the same time his brother Cecil left for Johannesburg, where he managed the Transvaal operation together with Neil's university friend Ray Hasson.

Joe was impressed by his sons' abilities 'after so few years of practical experience'. He told a friend, 'It's amazing, the decisions I come to after thirty years of practical experience, the boys arrive at too, with only five years of university training.'[101]

~

Never-ending dust … and running around barefoot. These are Neil Jowell's overriding memories of growing up in Springbok. 'And going to the garage, as it was then, to see my father.' As childhoods go, it was not a particularly happy one. But it was not unhappy either, he quickly points out. Yet 'nothing stands out'. As with Kate's childhood, there are hardly any stories to tell or anecdotes to recount. Neil has always had a good relationship with his brother Cecil, who is two years his junior, even though 'there was the usual rivalry when we were growing up'. Both Neil and Cecil were born in Cape Town, where Bessie's brother, Dr Harry Berelowitz, attended the births of both boys.

After Cecil was born, Joe and Bessie moved to a house they'd built on the main road, right on the edge of the village. Not only was it one of the last houses on the road out of Springbok, but it also defied expectation, as journalist Anneliese Kuhn discovered.

Kuhn flew to Springbok in a Namakwaland Lugdiens Piper Navajo, owned by Joe Jowell, the man she was due to profile for *Scope* magazine as part of a series on 'Men with Millions'. Kuhn expected to find 'a grand old homestead in the same tradition as the kind found dotted all over the Cape; white-washed, gabled, walled-in, plenty of yellow-wood, fine furniture, a brigade of servants …'

Instead, she found a simple, honest, if charmless, home: the sitting-room floor was covered by a shabby red-and-white carpet, the furniture had 'seen better days', the pictures on the wall hung carelessly askew, and one of the windows had a yellowing piece of paper stuck to it.

But then, she pointed out, 'you notice the grand piano, and that the lady of the house wears a large flawless diamond – and you become aware of the telephones. Their ringing punctuates the day from 6 am until late in the evening, with the calls going out and coming in from Johannesburg, Pretoria, Cape Town – making for a telephone bill of R1 000 a month. Telephones in the sitting room, dining room, bedroom and even in the bathroom-cum-lavatory – where Joe Jowell is said to prefer making his most important decisions. It becomes evident that, contrary to appearances, this is not an average drab little home – it is a powerhouse of big business.'[102]

Bessie would, in her no-nonsense way, later tell Anneliese Kuhn that 'possessions are a nuisance'. Joe, too, expressed distaste at being labelled a millionaire, deeming it to be an 'absolutely meaningless word'. Bessie added, 'We aren't millionaires. We don't live like millionaires. The whole idea is despicable with its connotations of playboy-ism and squandering money. We aren't like that.'

In spite of its modesty, the house was always humming. Joe and Bessie were great entertainers. Their parties – and there was more than one every week – were legendary.

Neil and Cecil attended the local Afrikaans primary school – only because Bessie would have it no other way. She dismissed the opinion of the principal, 'Oom Piet' van Heerden, that the boys should go to the English school at Okiep. 'Oom Piet' put up a fight, but he backed off when Bessie threatened to involve the Minister of Education if he refused to enrol her sons. Eventually he relented, and Neil and Cecil spent their primary school years at 'Oom Piet's school'.

During one interview, Neil refers to his report cards for Sub A, Sub B and Standard 1 (Grades 1, 2 and 3), which he has kept. 'I was fluent in Afrikaans because we were at the Afrikaans school – which was only about 100 metres from the house – and Springbok was very Afrikaans. In my first year at school I came fifteenth out of a class of thirty. I was absent a lot – I remember I had a problem with my joints and I couldn't walk properly. Anyway, by Sub B I had improved my position in the class – I came seventh, and in Standard 1 I came first.'

It was the beginning of an outstanding school career. After primary school, both boys were sent to an English high school in Cape Town, Wynberg Boys' High. Neil's high school career began at age eleven, as did Cecil's, two years later. Neil spent very little time in Springbok during those years, only returning home for the school holidays.

After matriculating, he went to UCT for five years, completing a BComm, followed by an LLB degree.

But Neil couldn't quite see himself practising as a lawyer, so he returned to Springbok to work in his father's business for three years. He spent the following year overseas, on a 'grand tour', before returning to Springbok in the mid-1950s for another stint at Trencor. By then he had married Bertha Hershler.

In the early 1960s, Neil and his young family – by this time Paul and David had been born – went to New York, where he did an MBA at Columbia University.

'It was fascinating being in the United States at that time,' he recalls. 'New York wasn't the dangerous place it would become in the late 1960s – the university is in Harlem, virtually on Broadway. But we were there during the Cuban missile crisis, and my father phoned and demanded that I come home – he didn't want us getting stuck there during a war!'

Neil's stint in London followed, after which he, Bertha and the boys returned to South Africa. 'By then Cecil was working in the business too, and it really was too small a business for the two of us, and I didn't want to go back to Springbok anyway. So I came to Cape Town to run a small part of the business here. I never lived in Springbok again.'

Today, Trencor's main business is the worldwide leasing of marine containers. Neil's working day is extensive, as he connects with his colleagues – based mainly in America – until late into the night. And whether he is working or not, Kate sticks close to him when he is at home, following him around, seeming to need his presence, if not his attention. My attempts to talk privately with Neil always end fairly soon, as Kate inevitably appears in the doorway, seeking us out, willing us to include her, it seems, in a world from which she is increasingly excluded.

But perhaps she is also determined to participate in the interviewing process of pinpointing the highs and lows of her life, to hold onto what she still can, to continue to shape her life, if only its written version.

From our earliest interviews, it is strikingly apparent that Neil is very proud of Kate's achievements – from the time of those dramatic days when he first met, and married, the poised and talented Kathy Bowman.

~

It was a low-key affair – on 8 October 1970 – at the Caxton Hall registry office in London. The bride wore a chic, deep-purple two-piece. The bridegroom was attired in a sober suit. 'I don't remember why we got married at Caxton Hall – though it was the place where many film stars got married at the time!' Neil says.

The light in the study falls sharply on his desk. Kate, sitting opposite him, listens intently, even though her face is, at times, devoid of expression. 'We were obviously not going to have a big wedding and it was as good a place as any. We used to go to London every year in September for two weeks.'

Neil's good friend Ray Hasson and his wife Sheila were on hand to witness the couple's big day. Neil confesses that the run-up to the event was marred by his quibbling over Kate's yen to buy a special outfit for the occasion.

'It was one of our biggest fallouts,' he says. 'A few days before the wedding – or was it after? – Kate wanted to buy a dress, and I said to her, "Why do you need a new dress and why do you want to pay so much for it?"'[103]

Kate shakes her head rather bemusedly. 'I don't recall any of it.' Neil continues. 'It must have been before the wedding because she obviously wanted the dress for the ceremony. I don't remember now whether she bought it or not ...' He turns to Kate and grins, 'You told me I was *snoep* (stingy)!' She laughs, a knowing look crossing her face. 'You cried at the registry office,' she offers suddenly. Neil questions the fact, but says with good humour, 'I won't deny it ... I am a soppy character!'

A week later, when Kate and I meet for a chat at Carlucci's, I ask her about the public response to her affair with Neil. Increasingly, I find myself using the phrase 'Do you remember …' as the opening gambit. It's a bad move on my part, for it serves to heighten the fact that, most days, she can't remember the details of her life story. There are moments that are more lucid than others, when her memory is clear and strong. But today, to one of my questions, she retorts with exasperation, 'I'm completely clueless. I'm trying to see what I can dredge out of my mind, but it's terribly foggy.'

I ask her about the outfit and how she felt about the argument. 'I can't remember it – but I must have said, "Well, I'm not getting married then" if he refused to pay for it. But he really did cry, and I think I was crying too … probably because he was so mean! What a man …'[104] She looks at me, then chuckles heartily.

But the marriage of Kate and Neil caused tension elsewhere. Kate's parents, George and Kathleen Bowman, who had moved to Cape Town from Bulawayo by then, were 'concerned about the situation'. Paul Bowman recalls, 'I remember well Kath's marriage to Neil. Everybody was concerned.'[105]

Neil's parents, Joe and Bessie Jowell, were more than concerned, however. 'They clearly didn't like the arrangement,' Neil recalls. 'My brother, Cecil, was fairly neutral about it, but my family clearly didn't like it. My parents were opposed to my relationship with Kate, and our subsequent marriage, but I didn't need, or ask, their permission before going ahead. They did try to dissuade me. The fact that Kate was not Jewish didn't really play a role. My mother was a rabbi's daughter, but my parents were not really very religious. My father was an integral part of the Jewish community, but his life extended way past that small community of twelve people.'

Yet, as a Jewish family, the Jowells pressurised their elder son not to end his fourteen-year marriage. 'Jewish families did that,' Neil remembers, 'but not directly. They put pressure on me through common friends, and through our attorney.'

But Neil went ahead, and paid a personal price. 'Divorce was a bit more unusual in 1970 than it is now,' he says ruefully, 'and it was personally a very difficult time. My sons were very upset when I left, and for the first few years things did not work out very well.'

At the time, Kate was not oblivious to the consequences of her marrying Neil. It is telling that she is able to reconstruct the events, even through her Alzheimer's haze.

'What happened was not right; I didn't feel good about it. But Neil was determined that we should be together. Though I suppose that does not mean that I didn't have a choice in the matter, does it?' She smiles enigmatically. She stares down, unseeing, at her empty cappuccino cup. She lifts it uncertainly to her mouth, but then lowers it again, battling to find the saucer, which offers no comfort.

And then she repeats, again, as if to wipe away the memory, 'I felt remorse about it.'

Whatever her feelings at the time, though, she had made a choice, and a new life, and a new decade, with fresh challenges, beckoned.

7

Editor

(1970–72)

ECEMBER 2002. I am a few minutes late. This is not what I'd
intended. Ideally, I'd have wanted to be the first to arrive at the
restaurant, to observe my lunch companions from the start. To glean,
perhaps, an insight, the kind that offers itself in an unconscious gesture.
As I drive, I think about the two women I am about to meet. Of the two,
I know one fairly well. The other I know of but have never met. I am
apprehensive, sensing from what I know – and don't know – that I will
come to know her as much by the facts of her life as by the sum of the
unconscious gestures, the particular language of her being.

I park my car in the upper reaches of Cape Town's central business
district and make for Heritage Square at a stride, thinking about the
formidable duo who are waiting for me. Both in their early sixties, these
women have had careers that collectively span more than eighty years.
For the past four decades they have forged inspiring career paths for
other women to follow. They have shattered the proverbial glass ceiling
with determination, a steely resolve, poise and dignity. Each one has made
a difference to the world of South African women.

As I enter the dimly lit restaurant, I see them immediately. Kate Jowell
and Jane Raphaely are seated next to each other, almost awkwardly,
sharing the same personal space. In the past, Kate and Jane – who have
known each other for nearly forty years – would have asserted their
presence differently. They would have mapped out their own territory,

independently of each other. Once, both were powerful and influential. Now, only Jane is still making her mark. Kate's contribution is over, unfairly nipped in the bud in 1999 when the diagnosis of probable Alzheimer's disease precipitated the end of her working life.

I have never before given Alzheimer's much thought. I've had no personal or professional encounter with the disease – until this hot, blustery December day. Kate is smartly dressed, but her emerald-green blazer is inappropriate in this warm weather. She keeps it on, all the same. It doesn't occur to me that, perhaps, the simple act of removing an item of clothing like a jacket is something she can no longer do.

Yet it is easy to forget how much we need to remember in order to do the simplest things. In his foreword to David Shenk's definitive work on the disease, *The Forgetting – Understanding Alzheimer's: A Biography of a Disease*, Adam Phillips explains: 'We don't think of ourselves as having to remember our own names, or where we live, or how to eat or read. And yet, memory – all the skills and impressions we so carefully acquired in the past – informs much of what we do.'[106]

Phillips points out that we know how to play a game when we are familiar with the rules. And because we know the rules, we don't have to think about remembering them. This is a sign of success – being able to do things without thinking. 'And we call this second nature, presumably, because we think of natural things, such as recognising your mother's face or knowing where to sleep as virtually automatic. It is only when things begin to go wrong that we begin to notice just what it is we have been taking for granted. Our incompetence is a revelation.'

The experience of forgetting brings home to us the significance of memory. 'Alzheimer's as a disease – and as a disease we should remember that it is as natural as the lives it so insidiously disrupts – reveals just how unforgiving forgetting can be. And just how dependent we are on our memory: and so, how dependent we are on others when we lose it.'[107]

Four years after her retirement, Kate Jowell can no longer go to a restaurant alone, order a meal, enjoy it and settle the bill. Yet she seems to accept this sobering fact, perhaps because it has been dulled by time.

When I am introduced to her, she is friendly but nervous, her right hand constantly searching for the lapel of her jacket. We begin to talk about her life, and she is open about the dread disease that has cut short her career at its zenith. Her voice is light and high, her laugh ready.

It's not immediately apparent that she is sick. You can't easily detect the extent of the problem – until you listen carefully to her as she unpacks her life, and you try to make sense of the higgledy-piggledy chronology she presents. Sometimes she admits, with a forced light-heartedness, that she has lost the thread.

Jane helps her story along. Later, she advises Kate on what to choose from the restaurant's menu. An easy-to-eat pasta with pesto. It dawns on me – and it is a terrible realisation – that this once independent, extraordinary woman can no longer use a knife and fork. She gets by with a spoon, but even then several tubes of wayward penne land messily on the tablecloth. She seems mortified, but bravely tries to hide her distress.

This inability to identify everyday objects – such as a knife and fork – and their uses is one of the most disabling manifestations of Alzheimer's disease. The medical term for it – agnosia – is derived from the Greek, and means 'without knowledge'. Agnosia is the reason for many of the bewildering behaviours seen in the disease, say doctors William Molloy and Paul Caldwell in *Alzheimer's Disease*.

So, for example, the look and feel of a knife and fork do not trigger an understanding of what the objects are or for what they are used. Molloy and Caldwell explain that the vision and touch of an Alzheimer's sufferer remain intact within the brain, but what has been damaged is the ability to put these sensory inputs together to form a concept of an object recognised as a fork or a knife.

'What we know is that certain areas of the brain are badly affected early in Alzheimer's disease, while others are relatively spared. Unfortunately, the pathways that link the brain's various centres are often damaged quickly, so that specific parts of the brain can no longer communicate with each other, even though they themselves may function relatively normally,' Molloy and Caldwell note. 'Much as our cities are interconnected by motorways, telephones, satellite hook-ups, so the various centres in the brain are interconnected through neural pathways that transmit information instantaneously. Thus, the speech centre in the left temporal lobe knows what the visual centre in the occipital lobe is "seeing" and what the emotional centre in the limbic system is "feeling".'[108]

When the pathways linking these centres are damaged, they are unable to receive input from, or to influence, one another. 'A man with Alzheimer's is given a fork, and his sensory centre recognises it as something he has seen before, but with the pathways damaged he cannot tell you the name of the object he is holding, and he has absolutely no idea what it's used for or how he should hold it.'[109]

Kate seems to know what the utensils are for, but she is at the stage where she doesn't know how to use them. Jane is clearly unsettled to see her friend in this terrible spiral. 'I saw her a month ago and she seems worse today,' she confides. Reflecting on the lunch some weeks later at her top-floor office at Associated Magazines, Jane says, 'You can't anticipate the moments of lucidity with someone who has Alzheimer's.'[110]

Alzheimer's is often referred to as a disease of 'insidious onset' because it has no definitive starting point, says David Shenk.[111] The plaques and tangles proliferate so slowly – over decades, perhaps – and so silently that their damage can be nearly impossible to detect until they have made considerable progress. It is an 'invisible, ever-shifting' illness.

I had first heard, in passing, that Kate Jowell had Alzheimer's disease about two years prior to meeting her. A mutual friend had revealed how Kate had arrived at a lunch dressed, inappropriately, in evening wear. In my mind's eye, it seemed a pitiful sight. At the time I knew who Kate was because her career moves and rise to the top had been well documented in the South African media.

Also, she had been listed as one of South Africa's leading women in the *Women's Directory*, which I had edited for *Femina* magazine in 1995 and 1996. I clearly remember Kate's entry and her photograph, even though the image was not used. And, of all the hundreds of guests who attended the 1995 *Directory*'s launch party – which became something of a society event – it is only Kate Jowell's arrival that has remained vivid in my memory. I can still see her walking up the stairs, beautiful and confident, her perfectly bobbed hair swinging about her face. Then she disappeared into the humming crowd to mingle, to take her place among her peers, a woman truly worthy of the accolade.

Revisiting, now, the *Women's Directory* entry of Professor Kate Jowell, I am aware that it has the brisk insufficiency that is often typical of such summaries, the whole always being more than the sum of the parts: Kate Jowell, the holder of two degrees, director of the University of Cape Town's Graduate School of Business, director of First National Bank (Western Cape), Sanlam and Cadbury Schweppes SA, labour mediator and a women whose expertise earned her a place on both the National Manpower Commission and the Margo Commission on tax.

The entry leaves a very clear impression of a capable achiever – yet, as I now attempt to document Kate's life, I am struck by a number of omissions. Possibly the most ironic of these is the absence of any mention of her two-year tenure, from 1970 to 1972, as editor of *Fair Lady*, a magazine that held powerful sway at the time and profoundly changed the way women – and their daughters – perceived themselves and their role in society.

~

'Special report on African nannies'. 'What the next year holds for Jackie Kennedy'. 'Do they spare the rod and spoil the child in our schools?' 'Portrait of an actress: Yvonne Bryceland'. These issues and personalities, highlighted on the covers of early *Fair Lady* magazines, would have been on Kate Jowell's mind. In 1970, after assisting Jane Raphaely as her deputy for six years, she took over as editor. Jane remained the editor-in-chief, but she took on two new Nasionale Pers magazines, first *Close Up* and then *Modern Woman*.

In Kate's capable hands, *Fair Lady* continued to flourish. Veteran journalist Lin Sampson credits Kate Jowell with kick-starting her extraordinary career. Lin joined *Fair Lady* as a secretary in 1970, after a working spell in Greece and 'a lifetime in London'.

'Kate was instrumental in getting me the job,' Lin recalls, 'and for the first few months I worked exclusively with her.' Lin made a favourable impression, and Kate recognised her writing potential early on. Before long, she became an editorial assistant. Lin has warm memories of her mentor.

'I really liked Kate; she was always very fair. She was an incredibly decent person, and a very, very clever one at that. I had huge respect for her, and I know a lot of other people did too. She had that logical, mathematical brain, which was very appealing, because she looked at things in a very clear way.'[112] Kate's image – her svelte form and newfound glamour, complete with sporty little car and clothes to match – didn't go unnoticed. 'I remember this very thin, very beautiful woman, who had a wonderful wardrobe and drove a sports car,' Lin says.

But there were elements of Kate's personality that jarred with this snappy, somewhat sexy image. At heart, she was not a free spirit. She tended to be 'schoolmarmy', something the staff joked about among themselves. 'A colleague once received her copy back from Kate with "9/10" written on it!' Lin chuckles. In retrospect, Lin says she sometimes found Kate quite difficult to talk to. 'She would often just stare at you; perhaps that was the start of the oddities in her head ...' And there were also the rumours of her relationship with Neil Jowell.

Fashion editor Sydney Baker, a hand-picked *Fair Lady* team member from the magazine's inception, recalls that though Kate never mentioned Neil to her colleagues, he often appeared at her side. 'Once we were going to the Canary Islands on assignment for *Fair Lady*, and he was at the boat to see her off. She didn't talk much about him, but she certainly seemed very happy with him.'

Sydney had witnessed Kate's intriguing post-Neil transformation. 'She was a changed person,' he says in a telephone call from his home just outside Athens, Greece. 'Her whole style and appearance had changed. She'd slimmed down – not that she was fat before, but she'd certainly been nicely rounded. *And* she started driving a red Fiat Herald. When she was living in Kildare Road, she really was a plain Jane.' (Flamboyant 'Sydders' – the name given to Sydney Baker by the irrepressible Gorry Bowes Taylor, and the one Kate still uses when she speaks of him – had a close, happy working relationship with 'Kathy'. 'She was very clever, and rather quiet. She was reserved, and as a result I think some people perceived her as being a bit stuck-up, but that was not the case. She was very pleasant, and she had a wonderful wit.'[113]

When Sydney Baker left *Fair Lady* after close on three decades, Kate attended his farewell function. In a book of tributes designed as a farewell gift, she recorded the two one-liners that, in her view, summed up 'Sydders'. The first, his standard advice when things were threatening to get out of hand: 'Never mind, ducky, just have a cup of tea and a lie-down.' And the second, voiced when she ventured into the office – clearly during her plain-Jane days – in an uninspiring outfit: 'Nice idea, dear. Pity it looks like it's been put together with a knife and fork!' Kate remembers Sydney's melodramatic retort with a laugh, and repeats it gleefully whenever we speak of her time at *Fair Lady*.

Sydney Baker's appointment was something of a coup for Jane Raphaely and *Fair Lady*. A native of the Eastern Cape, Sydney had fled its parochial climes at the earliest opportunity for London, where he trained as a dress designer at St Martin's College. After graduating, he landed a plum job with the great fashion house of Balenciaga in Madrid before returning to the British capital to gain further experience with famous English designer Norman Hartnell. 'They were the top designers of the 1950s, so I was very privileged to work for them,' Sydney recalls.

But his parents' ill-health prompted his premature return to South Africa, to Johannesburg, where he joined the *Rand Daily Mail* newspaper's fashion and features department. Through his work he met Jane Raphaely, who was in the advertising industry at the time. She was sufficiently impressed with Sydney to offer him a place on her elite team when she started *Fair Lady*. But the time was not right.

'I declined the offer at first because my parents were in Johannesburg and I didn't want to live in Cape Town. But then my brother was transferred to Cape Town and my parents decided to join him. I thought I may as well go, too ...'

It was the start of a remarkable twenty-nine-year association with the magazine. Sydney joined Jane and Kathy, Peggy Page – the first beauty editor who, like Sydney Baker and food editor Annette Kesler, became something of an institution at the magazine – and also Jeremy Laurence.

Sydney soon created a name for himself as *Fair Lady*'s fashion editor. 'Jane decided that the clothes we featured had to be affordable, and they had to be available in South Africa. Everyone worked around that concept, and it was such a success. The fashion we featured was beautiful. Kathy was devoted to the idea too, because for her everything had to make sense, the idea had to be logical.' The pair worked closely together, and, like others, Sydney remembers Kathy's no-nonsense reputation and her conscientious approach. 'But she had a good bit of wit, too,' he adds.

~

'I have a black belt in café chairs,' Kate says with characteristic good humour as she tries to hoist herself onto one of Carlucci's high stools. Most days, she needs some guidance. Usually, I manoeuvre her until she's facing the right way, then she finds the chair's metal footrests and is able to lift herself onto the seat. Today, however, we're battling. She can't figure out what she's supposed to do, or why. She understands that she has to sit down, and bends her knees to lower herself, but the seat of the stool is too high. Feelings of desperation and panic well up in me. The words I use to direct her seem meaningless. She is unable to translate my words into simple actions. I am acutely aware of the stares – some sympathetic, others simply curious – of other Carlucci patrons. Then, suddenly, Kate's done it. She's sitting down, facing the right way.

We have a rendezvous with Annette Kesler, who, with Gorry and Kate, is a member of the Capricorns' birthday triumvirate. Annette, with her dark, diva-like good looks, soon strides in. She is warm, friendly, talkative. At a time when many of Kate's friends and former colleagues are limiting their contact with her, Annette's attentiveness is welcome. Kate is happy to see her, and to relive her *Fair Lady* days through Annette's monologue. Very much the connoisseur, Annette rejects Carlucci's menu offerings and orders instead a toasted provolone cheese-and-tomato sandwich on 'good white bread', insisting that her sandwich be made with butter or olive oil, not margarine. This is the woman who, for more than three decades, has taught generations of South African women how to cook and eat. She still does, not from the pages of *Fair Lady* – she shed the magazine cookery editor's mantle in 1999 after thirty-one years – but from her cookery website.

Annette is generous in her praise of Kate Jowell and her influence. 'Kate was the most wonderful mentor,' Annette begins. 'She was there when I joined the magazine, and she was responsible for a lot of things. She was so creative, and she had broad horizons – she was international in her thinking – which I really appreciated. She was what I call an educated cook. There is a vast difference between the marshmallow-and-peppermint-crisp brigade and the Elizabeth David school. I am a purist, unashamedly, and Kate is too. She read a great deal, she knew about the good English cooks at the time – people like Elizabeth David and Jane Grigson.'[114]

But Kate was also a perfectionist and, after working with her for a short while, Annette adopted the same work ethic. 'One day we were photographing the food for one of the editions, and Kate took one look at the carrots and said, with mild disapproval, "Don't you think those carrots look phallic?" Then she turned her attention to the bread and said, "And that bread looks very dry" in the same tone of voice. Those kinds of things stay with you for the rest of your life,' Annette chuckles. Kate smiles, but doesn't comment.

On another occasion, the team was photographing a feature on fla-voured butters, and Kate, who was overseeing the shoot, was not happy with Annette's pair of butter pats. 'We were photographing the butters at my house in Milnerton, but Kate drove all the way to Rosebank to fetch her own butter pats for the shoot. She would go to great lengths until something was right. At the end of the day, her butter pats were not much better than mine, but she was going to make certain anyway.'

In the 1970s, when Annette started at *Fair Lady*, cooking for the freezer was in vogue. She wryly observes that many women who became converts after reading those articles 'are still obsessed with cooking for the freezer!' The arrival of blenders – which radically altered life in the kitchen – and nouvelle cuisine – with its meticulous plating of food – are two trends that stand out in Annette's memory.

But the essence of *Fair Lady*'s food philosophy was to 'keep things alive and innovative'. It was not formulaic. And it culminated in one of the magazine's first cookbooks, *Special Occasions*, which Kate and Annette jointly compiled. 'Two of the chapters, one on pasta, the other on after-theatre suppers, were shot by Desmond Bowes Taylor in Kate and Neil's new house in Glencoe Road. I remember the carpets were new, and Neil was very worried that we would mess on them!'

Though these were apparently happy times, Kate Jowell's tenure as *Fair Lady*'s editor was, in fact, drawing to a rather bitter close. Her once happy working association and friendship with *her* mentor, Jane Raphaely, was on tricky ground. After it became clear to Nasionale Pers that, in the thick of the 1970s recession, *Close Up* was not attracting advertising support, the company closed the magazine a year after its inception. *Modern Woman* was launched, but it suffered the same fate as *Close Up*. At some point in 1972, Jane then returned to her brainchild, *Fair Lady*,[115] and a battle for control ensued.

Neil Jowell succinctly sums up the situation by saying, 'After the other two magazines were closed, Jane came back to edit *Fair Lady* again and Kate said, "I'm running the ship."' He doesn't embellish on the incident. Instead, he simply says Jane's return caused conflict that was not resolved. And in any event, he maintains Kate was destined for greater things. 'She'd been at the magazine for about eight years, and I think she didn't find it that challenging any more. Clearly, she was interested in other things.'[116]

When I ask Kate about her fallout with Jane, she appears not to remember it. In an interview, she once said of her magazine years, 'I don't think it was really my métier, but I got totally absorbed in the job. There was something so satisfying to be in at the start of *Fair Lady*, and to watch it growing fat and beautiful.'[117]

Editing the magazine was 'a challenge', but eventually, as Kate later confided to Gorry Bowes Taylor, she 'felt cramped'. No doubt she did, and her journalistic career had run its course. But perhaps Kate Jowell is being her ever-discreet self. Clearly, being editor of South Africa's top women's magazine held some weight for her, for she didn't easily relinquish her hold on it when Jane returned to *Fair Lady*. Kate put up a fight, and the two clever, ambitious friends were suddenly rivals, and at daggers drawn. When the contest ended, with Kate resigning, it was the start of a long – and public – estrangement that would last nearly fifteen years.

Friends and colleagues have vivid memories of the debacle. Sydney Baker says 'the fallout between the two of them was very sad. When Jane came back to be editor instead of editor-in-chief, there was a lot of sadness. Naspers didn't take sides, but Kate decided that she was not going to put up with the situation, and for a long time the two were not on speaking terms. It was a classic power struggle. Kate was the editor, then suddenly she wasn't, but she went on to a much better career actually, a far more illustrious career.'[118]

Another former *Fair Lady* colleague says that the magazine staff were mortified, and 'didn't really know how to handle the situation, especially because they felt Kathy was treated shabbily'.[119] Kate's brother, Paul Bowman, concedes that 'it was a very bad time for Kath. Fortunately, she was able to rise above it.' Paul, then a senior executive with Johnson & Johnson International, finds it strange that a company like Nasionale Pers would 'change the roles of editors without properly and formally informing the persons concerned and those reporting to them'.[120]

Jenny le Roux also remembers the rift between the two women as being 'very bad' – and that Jane, too, was very upset about it all. 'But it must have been quite heavy because it went on for years, and as a result I didn't see Kate for a long time. In all the years that I have known Jane,

I have never known her to fall out with people. But it was a bad time for all concerned, even though we didn't really know what Kate thought about the matter.'[121]

Jane Raphaely is keen to tell the story, too. Far from shying away from it, or letting others tell it for her, it is almost the first thing she talks about when we meet in her spacious office, crammed with fascinating magazine memorabilia that document her rise to the top. 'Kate was the magazine's deputy editor, and then there was a period when she was editor and I was editor-in-chief,' she begins. 'Then I started two other magazines for Nasionale Pers. The first was *Close Up*, which was aimed at the youth market. It was successful as it had a high circulation, but we could not get advertising support for it. It eventually closed down after a year, and we started *Modern Woman* … Kate was not involved in either of these. Then *Modern Woman* folded, and I was asked by Naspers MD Dawid de Villiers to come back to *Fair Lady,* as the magazine's circulation and advertising support were shrinking. On my return I found that the system cut me off from having direct access to the rest of the staff. It didn't really work,' she muses.

Jane fixes me with an enigmatic stare and continues. 'We were not collaborating effectively. Kate resigned and went off to do something else.'

Of the fallout that would scar their friendship for many years, Jane says: 'We had been friends when I appointed her. But the eventual confrontation put a crimp in that for a while. We were estranged for a long time … and I remember exactly when we decided that this was stupid. We both belong to the 100 Club, and everyone in the club was extremely aware of the situation. One day, we were hosting a lunch at the old President Hotel in Sea Point. Everyone was seated and we were about to begin when Kate arrived. She was late. She came in, and the only vacant seat in the room was the one next to mine. Everyone froze, but I stood up and waved at her, indicating that there was a place next to me. She came over, sat down, and we started talking as if we'd never fallen out. It just shows how tough friendships really are, and what they can endure. If you don't care for someone, you would not react in that way,' Jane says.

On reflection, she cannot believe she was so 'stupid'. 'It's the only time in my life that I have been estranged from someone. I don't blame Kate for feeling whatever she felt when she resigned. But after the lunch, we just carried on as if nothing had happened.'[122]

It is indeed remarkable that their friendship not only survived, but began to flourish again after the 100 Club lunch. So much so that, at the suggestion of mutual friends, the Jowell family would later go on a Namibian camping holiday with the Raphaelys. Kate and Jane's ability to move on, to renew their bond, came at a time, in the mid-1980s, when they were both public figures, famous in their own right, confident of their ability and influence. In 1986 they would both be nominated by *The Star* newspaper as 'Women of Our Time' for their respective achievements.

But now Jane is the supportive friend as Kate battles to hold her own in any kind of company. Jane ensures that her friend is invited to birthday parties and other get-togethers, that she is not ostracised and forgotten simply because she has Alzheimer's disease.

∼

Jane, Kate and I are ready to leave the restaurant on Heritage Square. Clearly, Kate is tiring. We accompany her outside, and we watch her make her way haltingly across the uneven cobblestones to a waiting car. Rubin, one of Neil's Trencor employees, has come to take her home. Jane and I don't speak. We are lost in our own thoughts. It is nothing less than shocking to watch Kate, with her once-confident stride, struggling to walk two or three metres. The tiny cobblestones seem to turn into boulders in Kate's mind, and the few steps to the car door seem a perilous path.

Over our meal, we had spoken about the documenting of Kate's extraordinary life, the writing of a biography of a woman who has fallen prey to what Adam Phillips calls '*the* modern disease that, apart from cancer, haunts our lives',[123] a woman whose memory is being dismantled and who will regress and retreat into virtual infancy. The thought of this is chilling and horrifying, and as we wave goodbye to a smiling Kate, the image of her at the *Women's Directory* launch party comes back to me. For even then, in 1994, Kate Jowell's brain would almost certainly have fallen victim to the first incursions of Alzheimer's disease. This is a moment almost of foreboding for me, understanding as I do, after this first meeting, that the task I have been asked to undertake will be more than a process of dispassionate chronicling, and that growing close to an increasingly unknowable Kate will prove emotionally taxing.

I can barely imagine what it must be like for Neil Jowell. It is a measure of the strain he lives with that he finds it hard to control his emotions when, later, Jane calls him to talk about the book, and what the future holds for his wife, her friend.

part three

A BRAIN
FOR BUSINESS

8

MBA

(1973–74)

DURING HER EIGHT years at *Fair Lady*, Kate Jowell had 'learnt her trade as a woman'.[124] But when she turned her back on journalism, she was drawn once more to a male-orientated environment – the world of business.

In an interview in 1974, a year after leaving *Fair Lady*, she attributed her departure to needing to exercise her mind more rigorously; to grow in some new direction. 'I felt that I had always flitted. There had been no great depth. But I didn't want to start at the bottom of some new discipline.'[125]

She considered studying towards an MBA degree, 'a fast, one-year qualification, very measurable in a businessman's eyes', but she assumed it would be too demanding and that 'a lot of it would be rather tedious'. Then, the sudden death of her father-in-law, Joe Jowell, in January 1973 proved to be a turning point. 'My husband took over the company, which meant that he'd be very busy and less guilty about it if I was busy too ...'[126] In fact, Kate had never objected to Neil's work commitments. Which is just as well, for as Joe Jowell was known to tell his daughters-in-law, and also the wives of his employees, 'When you marry a transport man, you marry the business first, then the man.'[127]

At the time of Joe's death, Neil had been based in Cape Town. 'At that stage the Cape Town division of the business was a lot smaller than the operation in Springbok. When I took over as executive chairman of the Trencor group, I brought the head office to Cape Town,' Neil explains.

For Kate, it was a case of now or never as far as further study was concerned. She took the plunge, and it was a decision that both changed her life and set her career on a stellar course. That year, she was only one of a sprinkling of women to attempt the onerous postgraduate business degree at the University of Cape Town's Graduate School of Business. She stood out immediately. Not only because she was part of a small minority of women, but because she was intelligent, self-assured, articulate – and blessed with a natural grasp of business. 'Kate understood business very well,' Neil comments. 'She was very interested in it.' Then he adds, with a sudden spurt of humour, 'She was impressed by the shining example I set, and thought that if people of that calibre were in business, she would follow suit.'[128]

The MBA was demanding, 'pure slog ... a gruelling ten months with lectures six days a week and only brief breaks in between terms'. Kate worked eighty hours a week, she would later tell Gorry Bowes Taylor in an interview, wincing at the memory. 'Lectures every morning till 1 p.m. Nose down to my books at 2 p.m. Stopping to cook supper for Neil at 7 p.m. Back to my books at 8 p.m. and then up to the business school at 10 p.m. every night except Saturday for group meetings, which sometimes went on past midnight.'[129]

Detailing the rigours of the course, Kate continued: 'A group is six to eight people who meet for the whole year to help each other in various areas. You can't get through everything on your own.' Kate's MBA comprised sixteen courses, including Management Accounting, Statistics and Computers, Environment of Business, and Human Relationships and Organisation. The last of these, as she went on to reflect, was 'surprisingly a lot of what business is all about'.

Diligent and committed, Kate sailed through the year. 'You very early on devise a means of survival,' she explained. And in the business world, survival usually meant an ability 'to cut through one's work to the essentials at great speed'. Little wonder she excelled, with her ability to cut to the quick, to see things clearly, whatever the circumstances.

Her term paper was on consumerism. She was interested in marketing because so much of it was directed at women. 'I watch shopping-centre developments with great interest,' she revealed.

Her particular talents captured the attention of the Business School's director at the time, Professor Meyer Feldberg – currently a senior adviser at Morgan Stanley in New York City on leave of absence from Columbia University, where he is dean emeritus and professor of Leadership and Ethics at Columbia Business School. He was impressed, and long before she graduated he offered her a senior lectureship at the Business School. In a telephone interview from New York, he explains why Kate piqued his interest. 'In those days, most of the students were men. As a result, the women stood out. But Kate was very noticeable because she had presence, style and the intellectual capacity to lecture.'[130]

The appointment was a considerable achievement. The MBA environment is, by its nature, tough, competitive and ruthless. In this milieu, Kate showed her mettle. 'She was, and remained, a very articulate person,' Meyer Feldberg says. 'She spoke fluently, she spoke persuasively; she was passionate about things and issues that were important to her. This was crucial, because if you're going to be a teacher, you have to believe in what you're doing.'

In the midst of the hectic MBA year, Kate was also overseeing the building of her and Neil's first house. The couple had bought a plot in Gardens, right up against the flank of Table Mountain, in a little-inhabited cul-de-sac called Glencoe Road. It had spectacular views of Table Bay and the vast Atlantic, and the imposing mountain behind it.

The two-storey brick-and-timber house, with its wide wooden verandas, was built on the neighbouring plot of the home the Jowells live in today.

'Any five minutes I had off, I had to find floor tiles or chase a builder. And my July vac was spent moving into a house not yet finished, while my male colleagues played golf and relaxed,' Kate told Bowes Taylor. Four years later, the *Cape Times* included the house, which was built on stilts because of the steep terrain, in a series of articles on 'Colourful Cape Homes'.

In one of these articles, the feel and features of the Jowells' house were carefully described. The house reflected Kate's stylish touch, and the couple's interests. 'The house gets the sun from morning to mid-afternoon,' the article began, 'and colours are kept neutral to reflect the light. White-painted brick walls and natural woodwork make a perfect background for antique chests and many comfortable chairs in steel, canvas, wood and leather. The main living room doubles as sitting and music room. It has an unusual arrangement – a stainless steel fireplace set in the middle of a window wall. The windows have been brought as low as possible for maximum view, and one can enjoy a log fire as well as the sight of the city lights on winter evenings.

'Although the house is modern in style and there is a lot of glass, the materials are otherwise traditional. There are sloping timber ceilings with exposed beams and the floors are of gleaming brick, with heating from beneath.'[131] By all accounts, 48 Glencoe Road was a handsome home – cutting-edge and confident, though still warm and inviting.

But for a time, before and after their marriage, and while the first Glencoe Road house was being built, Kate and Neil lived in her cosy Rosebank cottage. It was there that Kate took the unexpected phone call from Springbok that would change their lives forever.

～

For Joe Jowell, the morning of 16 January 1973 dawned in the same way as any other. He was up long before dawn, and by 6 a.m. was already on the telephone, arranging meetings for later in the day. Thirty minutes later he was dead, having passed away in mid-sentence while talking to his wife, Bessie, about their plans for that evening. His relentless, self-imposed schedule, and the Stokes-Adams attacks he'd endured for more than twenty years, had brought his life to a premature close. He was only sixty-seven years old.[132]

It was the end of an era. Mourners descended on Springbok from all over South Africa. Thousands of people attended Joe's funeral – the largest in the history of Namaqualand. Phyllis Jowell recalls that the 'line of cars in the funeral procession was at times six kilometres long'.

With Joe's passing, life in Springbok and the Namaqualand region would never be the same. He had been associated with the town's phenomenal development for more than three decades, and was known as the 'Uncrowned King of Namaqualand'. From municipal affairs to keeping the Jewish community alive, to cultural and sporting matters, Joe's influence was wide-ranging. He had, as Rabbi Lapin observed in his funeral address, 'started off by linking Namaqualand with the rest of South Africa, and ended by linking Jew and non-Jew, family and friends, Springbok and other municipalities, South Africa and the international communities on which he served as a representative of his country'.[133]

In another tribute, Gordon Parker, an outstanding businessman who would become chairman of Newmont Mining in the United States, referred to Joe as 'a great son of South Africa ... a great son of Namaqualand'. He continued, 'We have lost a man of brilliant intellect. His keen and penetrating mind would cut through to the heart of the matter. We have lost a warm-hearted man. A treasured friend; a man of humour and generosity who loved people more than material things. He made friends – and these were deep friendships – with people from all walks of life. He knew both the rich and the powerful and the humble and the poor. They all beat a path to his door. But he never lost the common touch.'

Joe was a great giver, not only of money, but 'of time and heart', Parker said. Brave, gallant, determined, courageous. A man of honour and integrity. Joe's word was his bond, and everyone who did business with him knew it.

After forty-two years at the helm of his business, Joe had passed the stable, diverse, highly successful organisation he had built from scratch to his sons. Neil succeeded his father as executive chairman of Trencor, choosing not to continue the Jowell legacy in Namaqualand, but moving the headquarters to Cape Town.

~

April 2003. It is a mild Saturday morning, punctuated by strong bursts of wind. Kate and I make our usual way to Carlucci's, where we have a rendezvous with one of the first MBA students Kate taught at the Business School. South African–born Harris Gordon was a full-time student, a member of the 'Class of '73'. Quite by chance, just a week before, I had met his wife, photographer Tessa Frootko Gordon, at Vergelegen, a stately wine farm near Somerset West. We had sat next to one another at a function where Nelson Mandela addressed a grand gathering of eminent Rhodes scholars. Tessa was on assignment. I was a mere observer, in the right place at the right time – for, on hearing that I was working on a book with Emeritus Professor Kate Jowell, Tessa revealed that her husband had been one of Kate's first students, and that Kate had stayed with the couple in Boston during a visit some years earlier.

As usual, Carlucci's is abuzz. I steady Kate as she eagerly negotiates the sloping pavement and the tricky little step at the front entrance. Then the automatic doors whoosh open, ushering us inside. Harris and Tessa watch our unsteady advance. I can see that they are shocked at Kate's shuffle, at her excruciating battle to climb onto the high chair at this trendy suburban eatery. I order her usual decaf cappuccino and an Amsterdammer – the Dutch confection redolent with almonds that she so loves. I sugar her coffee, quarter her cake. Harris, particularly, must be trying to recall the dynamic, go-getting woman he had known and admired all those years ago. For the woman he sees before him today is not the Kate Jowell of his memory.

In the car, on the way to Carlucci's, Kate had confided that she did not, in fact, remember her former student or his wife. So it is left to Harris to fill in the gaps with snapshot images of their previous encounters. They are mostly of a young Kate trying to gain control of sixty-six rowdy, uncooperative men. He says to her that his MBA class had given her a hard time. She responds with humour. 'So you were nasty to me, were you? I don't believe it!' Kate considers the possibility, and then laughs. Earlier, Harris had confided that Kate, then a young and inexperienced lecturer, 'seemed to be having difficulties managing the class, and at some point a few of us had to intervene. We stood up and said, "Give her a break", as they were not paying attention.'[134]

Harris, a management consultant and retired partner at PriceWater-houseCoopers in Boston in the United States, tells me that Kate seemed to be quite distressed about the incident. For facing a roomful of MBA students is intimidating, concedes Harris, who teaches from time to time at Harvard University's Business School. 'It's like entering the lion's den!'

Kate has forgotten this ordeal, but she considers Harris's revelations and retorts, 'Oh, what a lot of clots you were! I've heard this stuff before, but I don't believe it for a moment.' She grins, then adds, 'Did you all think you were the bee's knees?'

Harris laughs. But it is hollow, not hearty. Kate's condition, which is certainly past the middle stages of Alzheimer's, has clearly knocked him off-centre. Kate, on the other hand, appears, for the moment at least, to have forgotten that she is a victim of the disease, her jocular manner seeming to suggest obliviousness to the evidence of its ravages.

In March 2003, just two months after meeting Kate, I tentatively raised the question of death and dying. Did she ever think about it; does it prey on her mind? 'No, I don't think about dying,' she replied, her eyes steadily meeting mine. 'I just think I'll fade away. One of the things that may kill me is cancer … but I don't think I'll get it now.'[135]

It is not unusual for Alzheimer's sufferers to be in denial. It is, in fact, 'an important part of the Alzheimer's experience', says David Shenk.[136] Denial 'is very commonly employed as symptoms first appear, or at the time of diagnosis, or at any juncture where a truth is so horrifying that the most emotionally healthy choice is to pretend that it does not exist,' Shenk goes on to explain. 'The poisonous reality is pushed back into the recesses of the mind and only slowly, in small drips, is it allowed to seep back into consciousness.'[137]

Mercifully, perhaps, the middle stages of Alzheimer's 'bring an end to ambiguity'. If before there were only subtle clues that something was amiss, there are now 'bright, self-reflecting signposts of decline, impossible to avoid'.[138]

The progression of Alzheimer's within the folds of the brain is marked by a precise trail of pathology. In the brain's hippocampus, the plaques and tangles have spread well beyond their starting points. Tens of millions of synapses have dissolved, disappeared. As the structures and substructures of the brain are so highly specialised, the exact location of the loss of neurons determines what specific abilities will be damaged, and when – 'like a series of circuit breakers in a large house flipping off one by one'.[139]

Memory formation fails. And once this happens, the person starts to lose control over primitive emotions, including anger, fear and craving. This often results in 'hostile eruptions' and 'bursts of anxiety'. Shenk describes the relentless domino effect of the ensuing damage: 'From there, tangles spread outward through much of the rest of the brain, following exactly the same pathways that sensory data travel in a healthy brain. One tangled neuron leads to another tangled neuron leads to another, like a pileup of cars after an accident.'[140]

~

Kate started her teaching career at the University of Cape Town Graduate School of Business by running two courses – 'the highly unpopular WAC – Written Analysis of Cases'[141] and Management in South Africa. Of the WAC course, she said in an interview, 'The aim is to develop [students'] analytical skills. Then there's the painful process of putting it down on paper. Everyone hates writing! But it does teach one to convey one's meaning crisply and concisely, which is basically what business reports are all about.'[142]

The management course was a forum in which top businesspeople, politicians and academics could share their expertise with the students. Kate was also responsible for grading the students' research papers, which dealt with different aspects of management in South Africa. 'Each paper runs from 10 000 to 20 000 words, which I then have to grade. Obviously I can't handle the paper if it's on too rarefied a subject, but the Business School has rich resources of experts that one can tap for this kind of aid,' she said.

It was a feather in her cap that she was responsible for the grading of the students' research papers. 'It was an important course,' Meyer Feldberg explains. 'You couldn't graduate without passing it.'

For Kate, the learning curve was steep, but she eagerly took on the challenge. Initially, her appointment was for one year, but in the first week of lecturing she confided that she would stay on if she were asked to. Though somewhat daunted at the new challenge of facing a class of highly critical graduate students, she was clearly in her element: 'I've enjoyed my work so far. My first lecture was only this week. That sea of sixty-six faces. It could be a success or it could be a total disaster!'

But it was not a disaster at all. Her new job may have had a scary start, but once again, with hard work, tenacity and a fine intellect, Kate Jowell rose to the top, the one-year appointment stretching to an impressive twenty-five-year tenure, with seven years spent as director of the Business School.

Ironically, at the start, she'd idly wondered how rewarding a career this would be. But she was soon keen to complete a doctorate. 'I feel I didn't get out of my MBA year as much as I should have done, as much as others did. There simply wasn't the time. We've an excellent library and I'm looking forward to exploring it.' Her instinct to study business served her well, even though she had certain reservations about the Business School – that some aspects would be boring, routine. 'But I've found it so creative … One forgets how much of business is people. It's not just books or selling widgets. It's a question of pricing, and the balancing of values,' she said. There were several elements of business that she found exhilarating.

Emeritus Professor John Simpson, currently the University of Cape Town's acting dean of Commerce, was deputy director of the Business School when Kate joined the teaching staff. He remembers that he and Meyer Feldberg spent a long time trying to identify an area of business that would interest Kate. He goes on to explain: 'She didn't come from a clear-cut business background. Most MBA students have business experience in a particular area, or they're professionals, like lawyers or engineers. Kate's undergraduate degree was in Applied Mathematics, which is remote when seen in this context.'

But it was Neil who finally pointed her in the right direction. 'At the time I could see that the union movement was gaining momentum and that industrial relations was going to dominate the business arena in the future. So she started taking an interest in labour affairs,'[143] Neil says.

John Simpson found Kate's affinity with industrial relations intriguing because she had indicated that sociology, economics and labour were not her fields, and she had to learn it all from scratch.[144] In time, she would come to know her field backwards, and soon she was acknowledged as one of South Africa's few industrial relations experts – and certainly the only woman expert in the field. Her gender would be an omnipresent factor, right up until the end of her career. When she started lecturing, there were no women doing the course. 'You must be motivated to write off a year of your life,' she said, explaining that married women 'don't always have the motivation – unmarried women can't easily drop a year's salary and shell out R1 000 for the course. The men who do the MBA are those who want to get further faster, to really move in management. One of the problems about being the only woman here is that you tend to be viewed as a spokesperson for women in general. And then you tend to think of yourself as such. Which, of course, I'm not. I suppose I'm a bit of an oddity.'

Kate was, assuredly, a singular woman with singular talents. In a decade in which women in developed countries all over the world were objecting to the glass ceiling, Kate Jowell was a pioneer in becoming a leader in what had always been a man's world.

9

Motherhood and More

(1975–79)

'SHE POSSESSES A rare instinct, one that allows her to recognise change at its inception. Kate is not the kind who makes waves; her true genius lies in knowing how to ride them.'[145]

This observation regarding Kate Jowell's character would prove true throughout her rise to the top – both as a business academic and as an industrial relations expert. She had found her niche, and the timing was impeccable.

The 1970s ushered in a new, dramatic phase in South Africa's labour history. The dynamics and the policy shifts of the period went to the heart of what was – in the rhetoric of the time – the 'arena of struggle'. Kate Jowell both foresaw and understood this. In sharing that understanding, always with optimism and self-assurance, she became, in a sense, an agent of change. She knew South Africa would never be the same again after the events of the early 1970s, and she participated constructively in the transition.

For almost a century, as noted in *Every Step of the Way*, 'cheap black labour had … been the mainstay of white well-being and wealth, and good returns for international investors. It was a pattern established in the early days of diamond and gold mining in Kimberley and Johannesburg in the last decades of the nineteenth century.'[146]

South Africa's industrial relations system did not allow for the expression of conflicting views, and there were no mechanisms for conflict resolution. One of the key labour laws of the apartheid era, the Industrial Conciliation Act of 1956, excluded blacks from its definition of an employee. This meant that black workers were barred from registered trade unions.

Yet, despite the illegality of industrial action, in 1973 a series of often violent wildcat strikes hit Natal, various parts of the Rand and the Eastern Cape. These involved up to 200 000 people, signalling that black workers were ready to use their collective strength to demonstrate rising intolerance of the status quo. The government met this show of militancy by strengthening the old Bantu Labour Settlement of Disputes Act of 1953, which had provided for limited communication channels between blacks and their employers. The revised law became known as the Bantu Labour Relations Amendment Act of 1953, and it encouraged employers to establish committees of workers as an alternative to unions. But, in the interests of productivity and foreign investment, employers started to urge the government 'to consider including Africans in the industrial relations process'.[147]

Towards the end of the 1970s, two commissions were appointed to look into labour questions, 'with far-reaching and unforeseen consequences'.[148] The Wiehahn Commission, under Professor Nic Wiehahn, convinced parliament in 1979 to extend labour legislation to African workers. It pointed out that the continued exclusion of black workers from recognised trade union membership 'was not only socially unjust but it could also lead to undesirable consequences of which industrial unrest was the least'.[149]

In the course of the next six years, the Wiehahn Commission reforms gave 'immense political leverage to hundreds of thousands of black union members who used it to press for both workplace and socio-political rights. This was especially so after the formation of the half-a-million strong Congress of South African Trade Unions in 1985.'[150]

The second government-appointed commission – the Riekert Commission, under Dr Piet Riekert – 'concentrated on ways to improve the quality and productivity of manpower and on various laws which also affect the optimal use of people and bring about regional settlement'.[151]

These labour reforms were the most exciting thing Kate Jowell had witnessed in South Africa, she declared in an interview a few years later.[152] She went on to explain that she had been in South Africa during a period of increased repression and polarisation, and she experienced 1979 as a watershed. 'Suddenly, one of the planks on which apartheid rested was simply pulled out! I could hardly believe it when I saw it happen, but it was exciting because it made possible an accommodation, a getting together, of blacks and whites in one arena.'[153]

At the time, Kate was establishing a firm reputation with her pioneering work in the labour arena. She may well have been 'a bit of an oddity', but as a stylish young woman with a grasp of complex, male-dominated fields, she attracted admiring attention. However, her position at what was then a 'white' university's Business School, and her marriage into the wealthy Jowell family, also burdened her with a 'white-elitist image that moved those in the labour movement to label her the academic mouthpiece for management'.[154]

Undaunted, Kate nevertheless worked hard to gain credibility as an impartial labour expert and consultant. Slowly, she reaped the rewards. In 1978 she was invited to speak at a prestigious international futures study conference in Grahamstown titled 'The Road Ahead', which grappled with the problems and challenges likely to confront humankind in the twenty-first century. Kate was in the news again the following year, when, with Professor John Simpson – then acting director of the Business School and deputy dean of the Commerce Faculty – she co-wrote a ground-breaking business management textbook, *Cases in South African Business Management*.

Aimed at students at universities, business schools and management colleges, the book was the first business management textbook to discuss and analyse South African case studies. 'Although many principles in business management are universal, there are areas in this country where, because of the environment, because of legislation and cultural values peculiar to us, the business manager faces problems that are unique,' Kate explained in an interview.[155]

The book was well received. *Finance Week* said it deserved 'a large readership', and praised the authors for providing a 'much-needed addition to a meagre South African management library and a first contribution to the finance and quantitative management case areas'.[156] The reviewer noted that Kate and John Simpson had 'successfully avoided the pitfalls of too little information for meaningful analysis, too much information resulting from hindsight and too direct information resulting from their own perception of the problem'.[157]

John Simpson explains that at the time there were very few case studies being published in South Africa. 'So we thought, if you took a typical MBA programme, you wouldn't really need ten case studies in each discipline, you would only need four or five. I recognised Kate's ability as a journalist and I thought her skills would be very useful. So we set about gathering material from colleagues.'[158]

For nearly three years, unsuspecting students analysed and resolved cases in the book, which were all tested 'as loose handouts, for their efficacy as teaching vehicles in either John or Kate's classes or those of helpful colleagues'.[159]

The book presents thirty-nine case studies in six functional management fields, including Marketing Management, Human Relations and Organisational Behaviour, Quantitative Methods in Management, Manpower Development, Financial Management and Business Policy. John Simpson wrote the majority of the case studies. 'Kate had a great deal to do with putting them together into a very readable format,' he says. 'She had a very clear mind, was very focused, and was a very good writer and editor. When she cut this book to pieces, it was a joy to watch.'

And occasionally, when he asked Kate to cast an eye over his 'painfully constructed' Chairman's Reports or speeches, Neil Jowell would also watch in awe as his creations assumed a new life and vitality thanks to her.[160]

Kate soon became a sought-after speaker at seminars and business functions, but the turning point in her career came later that year when she delivered a paper, 'Labour Policy in South Africa', to the Economic Society of South Africa.[161] Among the audience that evening was the respected economist Hennie Reynders, who was, at the time, also a popular candidate for many of the government's commissions.

'He was impressed by Kate's brilliance and recommended her to the Minister of Manpower Utilisation, Fanie Botha, who proposed her as a likely candidate for the Manpower Commission to Professor Nic Wiehahn, architect of revolutionary new labour policies for the country.'[162]

Kate Jowell's paper offers a clear and authoritative analysis of South Africa's volatile labour situation at the time. Commenting on the general state of affairs and the impact of the two commissions, she notes, 'One would need a literary talent well beyond mine to convey accurately the impact the Wiehahn and Riekert commissions and subsequent events have had on our country this year. We have seen euphoria. We have seen anger. We have seen disillusion and hope – a whole gamut of responses across every level of our society. If I must position myself on this spectrum – as I suppose I must – I would say my dominant emotion now is hope. And I don't believe I need to apologise for talking about emotions in this context and at this gathering, because subjective judgments are going to be major influences on how our labour policy and our future unfolds.'[163]

Kate's optimism was fuelled by the government's broad acceptance of the Wiehahn Commission recommendations, which represented, in her view, 'the most radical departure from accepted political and social practices in the past twenty years'.[164] She argued that 'government has acknowledged the equality of blacks as workers – both in their rights to trade union membership and in their rights to training and opportunity … the Riekert Report has also attacked discrimination in the workplace and laid the foundation for greater freedom and equality of opportunity for blacks – the central core of South Africa, at least'.[165]

Kate then went on to examine influx control and the associated policy of decentralisation. The former was the cornerstone of grand apartheid, which determined the residential status of blacks, as well as their geographic mobility. Scrutinising the Riekert recommendations on the infamous practice, she found one of the report's most 'difficult' weaknesses was its suggestion that the system should be retained.

She fearlessly communicated her opinions on the matter: 'I question on what basis it is more desirable to maintain the unemployed in the rural areas.'[166] But she also argued with fairness and lucidity: 'I would imagine there are strong economic arguments to suggest that to free the limits on the influx of blacks to our cities, to remove the restraints on their employment and training, would probably depress wage rates, would create over-crowding – but might in the long run lead to a more productive use of our resources.'[167]

The dismantling of influx control laws would, she believed, not only stimulate economic growth, but also accelerate the process of solving South Africa's social problems.

Kate's views on social and economic justice come through crisply and clearly. 'If the government is truly committed to hastening black access to the free enterprise economy as a means of capturing their hearts and minds – as well as, of course, a means of developing South Africa to its maximum potential – then blacks must see that that access comes without strings.'[168]

At the time, blatant discrimination continued, as blacks did not have the freedom to join trade unions, or to seek work areas of choice in their own country. 'Reasonable, patient people might argue that this is a temporary stage in the path to the orderly and gradual change we so desperately seek – but there may be few reasonable and patient people outside our own elite middle-class group. Not only may they fail to be reasonable and patient, they may be cynical and past the point of compromise.'[169]

Referring to the bloody Soweto uprising of 1976, when riot police ruthlessly opened fire on 10 000 marching schoolchildren protesting against being taught in Afrikaans, Kate warned that while 'large sections of our peoples neither have the vote, nor belong to formalised pressure groups … they have great informal power as the events of Soweto showed'.[170] She went on to observe that the country's social and economic institutions were so complicated that civil disobedience of a significant group can have 'disastrous consequences'.[171]

She concluded her address to the Economic Society on a cautiously positive note, saying that it was not too late to 'pick up the pieces', to 'repair the damage': 'I believe that to seek actively the views of all the corporate interests in our society, to be flexible in acknowledging and accommodating those views – and to be perceived to be doing so – will go some way to overcoming the problems of reforming and developing our industrial relations framework and, above all, of securing the commitment of everyone to making it work.'[172]

On another occasion – this time as guest speaker at a conference hosted by the South African Institute of Management – Kate spoke frankly of management's responsibility to resolve conflict in the workplace. 'The environment is becoming increasingly more conflict prone because of rising expectations on the part of blacks and because of job insecurity on the part of whites,' she warned.[173]

She said she had no idea how many companies operated formal grievance systems, though she did know that 'well under a million blacks are represented through liaison or works committees and around 70 000 through trade unions', this despite the fact that there were seven million economically active blacks in South Africa. In the future, she predicted, management would not just consult, but would also have to learn to negotiate with its workers because it had a 'wider responsibility to ensure that we have the maximum opportunity to maintain industrial peace in this country'.[174]

Soon after this address, and in spite of – or perhaps because of – her outspoken political views, Kate Jowell was among the forty-one prominent labour experts hand-picked by Minister Fanie Botha to serve on the National Manpower Commission for a two-year period. This appointment was a public acknowledgement of her skill and largely self-taught expertise – and it provided her with an extraordinary opportunity to help shape an evolving labour policy that would, eventually, have far-reaching effects. The minister made it clear that the government was waking up to the importance of labour matters, especially 'considering the significance thereof for the economic development and growth of our country and for the maintenance of sound human relations'.[175]

Members of the commission were selected for their expertise and experience, he added – though, in keeping with the times, he made no comment on the fact that the women commissioners were vastly outnumbered by their male counterparts. Kate Jowell was one of only two women in the line-up, the other being Lucy Mvubelo, general secretary of the National Union of Clothing Workers.

The appointment of the women provoked a mixed reaction. Most women's groups were grateful that they were represented, but, as *The Star* observed, 'women were not catered for in proportion to their working numbers' despite the fact that they constituted one third of South Africa's labour force.[176] Margaret Lessing, then a top businesswoman, tellingly acknowledged that, while she would have welcomed more women on the commission, 'the quality is there. These two women were chosen not because they are women, but because they are outstanding.'[177]

But Christiane Duval, who was a legal and labour adviser to the Johannesburg Chamber of Commerce, complained that 'once again women would have to make representation from the outside, not the inside', as Kate Jowell and Lucy Mvubelo had 'their own particular interests'. Duval's concern was the interests of working women that would, once again, be represented by 'the white male'.[178]

Kate, keen to be acknowledged as a person in her own right rather than as a token female, responded by stating that she did not represent any women's groups. 'I have probably been appointed because of my work in industrial relations and manpower development. I don't consider myself an expert on women in the labour force.' But she added that it would be a mistake to assume that because there were only two women on the commission, women's interests wouldn't be represented.[179]

In an interview soon afterwards, Kate explained that the National Manpower Commission was an advisory and investigative body recommended by the Wiehahn Commission to advise the minister on all labour matters concerning government labour policy and on all labour administrative matters. 'It will carry out investigations at its own initiative and also those referred to it by the minister.'[180]

When the interviewer, her old friend Gorry Bowes Taylor, pressed her on whether more women should have been appointed to the commission, Kate retorted, 'Well, it's 200 per cent more women than there were on the Wiehahn Commission. I don't know how the 41 members were decided on ... with me they've combined the interests of management education, industrial relations and women. With Mrs Mvubelo, they've got black interests, women's interests and trade unions. A 200 per cent improvement is a step in the right direction, isn't it?'[181]

The cool logic of her reply is revealing in a national climate of heated emotion. Kate Jowell, though a trailblazer, was not influenced by incendiary rhetoric: she was dispassionate in her approach, and this strategic wisdom would prove invaluable as her career status grew.

While Kate seemed impatient with suggestions that her inclusion had been motivated by the fact that she was a woman – albeit a knowledgeable one – she was, nevertheless, outspoken on the subject of women's rights and the bias against working women. Her views on the subject received considerable press attention when she addressed a Johannesburg seminar of the Secretaries' Club later that year.

Appraising the gathering, she launched into an argument about gender roles in modern industrial society: while the difference between masculine and feminine roles had been exaggerated, an increasing number of women worked for the same reasons that men did – to earn money or to pursue a career. These women were diligent and motivated, but were not getting the same rewards, the same opportunities or the same consideration as men in the workplace. 'You have probably seen advertisements for a lady accountant. That often means the company is looking for someone reliable, qualified and cheap, who won't want promotion.'[182]

Businesswomen were not a rare species, but very few made it to the executive suite. 'We are outnumbered in management, and it is at this level that the stereotypes are most prolific,' she continued.[183] Society maintained a rigid business structure, expecting women to adapt to an environment designed for men, by men. But women wanted their working environment to be redesigned to suit their own specific needs – and the changing circumstances in their lives. 'Working women are seen to be shy of taking responsibility, but this is often nothing more than the sensible realisation that, at certain times in our lives, we cannot take on any more, that we do not have the emotional energy to take on more demanding work because of our responsibilities at home and to our children,' Kate argued, continuing in her measured way, 'I believe that most women do not wish – contrary to the more radical view of the women's liberationists – to minimise their sexual and feminine roles as wives and mothers.'[184]

Kate's comments here, spoken from the heart in 1979, carried an added poignancy. For while her career gained momentum in the late 1970s, there were equally dramatic developments in her private life. She would soon embark on another, parallel course, one that would prove uniquely demanding, bewildering, enriching and rewarding: motherhood.

∼

May 2003. They have a lambency, a natural loveliness, about them, the Jowell daughters, Justine and Nicola, with their ready smiles and un-assuming manner, their apparent ease with their privileged place in the world. Photographs of the pair are scattered throughout the Glencoe Road house. The black-and-white portraits, which depict two little imps smiling benignly at the camera, arms flung around each other, are especially affecting.

When Kate married Neil in 1970, she was very keen to have children, to become a mother. 'I didn't really mind if they were boys or girls ... but I knew that I wanted to have children. I think Neil was ambivalent about it, but I insisted,' she remembers. At no point, however, did she consider giving up her newfound success in academia. She worked long and hard during both pregnancies, right up until the very last days.

When the girls were born, Neil was delighted. 'I was very pleased to have daughters,' he confirms.[185] Justine's dramatic arrival, on 17 July 1975, is still clear in his mind: 'The night before she was born, I was in Johan-nesburg on business. I flew back to Cape Town, and on arriving, I went to play a league squash game – I have always been a keen squash player,' he explains. 'Kate's gynaecologist was on leave at the time, and he was expecting to do the delivery on his return but he gave Kate the name and telephone number of the locum doctor. When I returned home after my game, at about 10 p.m., Kate was already in bed. I had to make an overseas phone call, and while I was talking on the phone, she suddenly said, "Don't talk for too long because my waters have just broken!"'

In a panic, Neil put down the telephone to attend to Kate. She contacted the doctor, who advised her to rush to the Vincent Pallotti Hospital in Pinelands immediately. But, true to form, Kate had other plans. She had been at work that afternoon, and insisted that Neil first drive her to the Business School so that she could tie up several loose ends before she was admitted to hospital.

'I was exhausted!' he recalls. 'I sat on the floor in her office, waiting for her to finish her work. Eventually I fell asleep. She was very focused, and an hour later we finally arrived at the hospital, to be met by a frantic doctor who was pacing up and down nervously awaiting our arrival.'[186]

Neil, who by his own admission is fairly squeamish, was at Kate's side throughout her labour and the eventual natural birth of his first daughter. 'I held Kate's hand, although I was probably looking away most of the time!' he jokes.

The arrival of a baby in the Jowell household had very little bearing on Kate's career focus. She enlisted the help of a nanny to care for Justine while she was at work. From the time of her marriage, she had also taken on the often rather awkward role of stepmother to Neil's young sons, who sometimes stayed at Glencoe Road at weekends.

'There was not that much contact between them and Kate in the early years after my divorce and remarriage,' Neil points out. 'But they did stay with us at weekends, and Kate, who was very precise and ordered, had to lower her standards somewhat when they were around, especially when it came to feeding them!' The boys seem to have accepted Kate's presence in their lives without too many problems. But, as Neil points out, Kate 'was not very demanding about being accepted' by the boys. 'It's just her nature,' he says, pinpointing an essential aspect of her personality.[187]

When Justine was three, Kate gave birth to another daughter. Nicola was born at Somerset Hospital on 5 January 1978. Though Neil was away on business at the time, he was, naturally, thrilled to hear of the birth of his second baby daughter. Today, his girls are confident, open-minded and free-spirited. And they are remarkably unencumbered by their parents' worldly success, which is, in equal part, a measure of their sure sense of self and the way Neil and Kate raised them. Kate was principled about money to the point of being Calvinistic, Neil notes. 'She was not materialistic and didn't expect handouts – and she instilled this attitude to money in the girls from a young age.' Yet their childhood was not without complications and compromises.

Life at 48 Glencoe Road was extraordinarily busy. Kate conceded, in 1979, that her work commitments the previous year – during which time the book she had co-authored was finalised for publication – had been onerous. Even Neil, who was very supportive, found her workload 'a bit much', she said.[188] Nicola was a newborn. Justine was a three-year-old toddler. And Kate had taken only four weeks' maternity leave after Nicola's birth. 'It was not long enough, the second time around,' she mused with some regret.

Yet, barely ten months later, Kate accepted the appointment to serve on the National Manpower Commission, which held its meetings in Pretoria at least four times a year. She must surely have been torn, leaving her little ones at home with a nanny, but the compulsion to excel at her career, to take up the opportunities that came her way, clearly proved too great.

The children would have felt her absence keenly, Nicola perhaps more so than Justine. The copious and colourful notes she wrote to her mother reveal an anguished little soul. 'Please don't go away again, Mommy. I'm scared when you're not here,' one of them reads.

Nicola, who left South Africa temporarily in 2002 to live and work in the United Kingdom, recalls that even though she wrote 'I'm-angry-with-you' notes to Kate throughout her childhood, she has, in fact, always enjoyed a good relationship with her mother. 'If I had a problem, I would always go to her, not to Pa.'[189]

Intense sibling rivalry with Justine marked her childhood. 'Though my parents were good parents and very fair, I always felt that Justine got more attention. I didn't like being the younger sister. Ma referred to it as my "counting things up": Justine did this, Justine did that. She was older, so, naturally, some things came to her first. I took my rivalry with Justine out on my mom because Pa was more aloof. It was always me and Mom. I wrote her notes from the time I was seven to the age of twelve. She kept all of them! Now I find them scattered around the house, which is a bit alarming.'

Justine, who in 2003 lives in Vredehoek and is a programme facilitator at Educo, a non-governmental organisation that works with disadvantaged youth, clearly remembers the rivalry. 'We fought quite a lot from early adolescence … we got on one another's nerves. I can't remember how Ma dealt with it. We had nannies who looked after us when she was at work or away from home. They were great, but in retrospect I would have liked her to have been there more when we were growing up.'[190]

But Justine does concede, with her ready smile, that the one advantageous aspect of Kate's regular travels was that she was often not around to sign the girls' homework books!

Even though Kate was a loving mother, the Jowell family was not openly affectionate. Nicola, who bears a striking physical resemblance to Joe Jowell, the grandfather she never met, says, 'We used to joke about the fact that whenever Ma came home and asked me how I was, I would always reply, "Fine." She worked hard and travelled a lot. I don't think I resented it, but I did miss her.'[191]

And when Kate was at home, 'she was always working' too. 'My dad used to take us to school in the morning, and one of the drivers from Trencor would fetch us,' Nicola says, describing a normal school day in the girls' early years. 'Our parents usually came home at about 6 p.m., and we'd eat dinner at about 7 p.m. Then they would watch the news on TV and, at 8.30 p.m. head off to their study to work.'

The girls went to bed, or did their own thing, as Nicola puts it. Kate was not only balancing the demands of two small children with those of what was by now an extremely exacting career, but she also had a household to run and commitments to a hard-working husband.

Before the arrival of the girls, Neil and Kate had regularly undertaken canoeing trips to the remote areas of the Orange River. The two of them were, in fact, early pioneers of river rafting on that part of the river – which has since become a popular contemporary activity. Neil believes: 'It was uncharted territory at that stage, and, apart from a trip by army personnel many years prior to this, no one had ever done anything like that before. In 1972, we did a six-day trip with some friends of ours, and for all that time we didn't see another person or any animals – apart from birds. It was extraordinary.'[192]

One of the friends who joined them that year, and several years afterwards on similar expeditions, was Jannie Graaff, eminent Cape Town economist and younger brother of the late Sir De Villiers Graaff. 'Neil initiated the trips through his Springbok connections,' Jannie says. 'We would drive to Springbok, park our cars at old Mrs Jowell's house in town, and a truck from Jowells Transport would then take us down to the river and dump us in with our canoes. Six days later, the truck would pick us up at what is now the Richtersveld National Park.'

Jannie, who would serve on a government tax commission with Kate a few years later, remembers her as 'a lovely person'. 'Kate not only supplied the food, but was cook-in-chief as well,' he recalls.[193]

Inevitably, the river-rafting expeditions gradually dwindled, and then finally stopped, once Justine and Nicola arrived. 'In 1980 we took Felix Unite on a trip, and he then commercialised river rafting. We were so used to being out on the river on our own, and once you've done it that way, if you encounter anyone else on the river, it spoils it for you,' Neil says.[194]

Kate enjoyed the trips, even though it was 'often quite frightening negotiating the rapids'. On one trip she lost her glasses, Neil recalls with wry amusement, and could hardly see what was going on. But there was no turning back. Kate carried on, uncomplaining and undeterred.

～

Kate managed her busy life by planning things meticulously, down to her supermarket shopping lists. 'I have a detailed checklist at home of the things we eat and use, listed as they are stocked on the supermarket shelves,' Kate once revealed in an interview.[195]

Then, of course, there were the Glencoe Road dinner parties. The Jowells entertained friends and colleagues with aplomb. Kate, who had retained her interest in food from her *Fair Lady* days, didn't blanch at all at the prospect of hosting a sit-down dinner for twenty people. Only on rare occasions would she enlist the services of a waiter or caterers, as she once did when hosting the Rhodesian Interim Government joint leader, Chief Jeremiah Chirau – one of three Africans who shared executive power with Ian Smith in the country's first step towards majority rule. Kate does not recall her father's reaction to her entertaining Chief Chirau: by then, after twenty-eight years, George and Kathleen Bowman had left their adopted country for good and had settled in Devon in the United Kingdom.

As in most areas of Kate's life, she was focused and thorough in her preparations for dinner parties. In a small navy-blue box, she recorded on index cards, in alphabetical order, the names of her guests, the dates of their visits, the menus on each occasion, and interesting snippets of information – whether about their culinary likes and dislikes, or their lives – that she wished to recall.

Caviar pancakes, saddle of lamb with red cabbage, and a maple parfait were on the menu when Business School director Meyer Feldberg and his wife Barbara dined at Glencoe Road on 8 August 1974. Other guests that evening included Anna Starcke and 'the Tebbits'. Jennifer and Hugh Herman were 'latecomers', Kate noted in another entry. 'She likes vodka or cane.'

'He is allergic to uncooked garlic and onion,' Kate wrote of another guest. 'Charles is their son,' she reminded herself of the Bowes Taylors.

The Galombiks, Yvonne and Arnold, were regulars over the years. Arnold, a prominent Cape Town attorney, was Joe Jowell's legal adviser and friend for years, and a director of Trencor until his death. Details of their visits fill several cards. On 20 October 1974, Kate served carrot soup, stuffed veal, and maple parfait. On 24 May 1979, guests sat down to mushroom soup, kabeljou, and brandy cake.

'The dinner parties were very elegant,' Yvonne Galombik recalls with pleasure. 'The Jowells were very hospitable, and Kate's food was delicious, and always beautifully served. The menus were interesting, the wine was good.'[196]

Flipping through the cards – the entries, a veritable who's who of eligible guests, stretch over a two-decade period – is a fascinating, revealing exercise. Kate's wit, her perceptive eye and her penchant for detail are clearly evident. 'He was overbearing,' she noted of one guest. Others had to endure 'overdone fillet'. And so on. Clearly, Kate was in her element during this period. 'I wouldn't change my life one iota,' she told Gorry Bowes Taylor. 'It couldn't be happier and fuller.'[197]

~

May 2003. I arrive at Glencoe Road to find Kate sitting in her favourite chair. Lately, she has taken to listening to the radio, which either Eunice Mzondi – Kate's ebullient housekeeper who has become her caregiver – or Vuvu, Eunice's daughter, has switched on for her. The sound is unbearably loud. Kate is staring blankly into the distance, unhearing, unseeing. As usual, the morning papers, still crisply folded, lie on the coffee table. She has ignored them for the past few weeks, even though a fresh batch is placed on the table every morning. For while Kate can still recognise certain individual words, she is no longer able to piece together an entire sentence.

I greet her cheerily, and she starts, as if she's snapped back suddenly from some secret distraction. Then, just as suddenly, she recognises me, and her face lights up. Her smile is radiant. 'Are we going for a cappuccino?' she asks immediately, trying to get up. She seems desperate to escape the confines of a house that has become her prison. Vuvu homes in on her when she hears we are heading for Carlucci's. 'Mrs Jowell, do you need to go to the toilet first?'

Kate ignores her.

'I need to speak to you,' she says to me, pushing past Vuvu. We negotiate, slowly and unsurely, the steep staircase to the street level of the house. In the car she says, 'No one understands that I don't ever pass water,' she begins. 'I don't know why that is, but I don't need to go to the toilet.'

I am startled. This is the first time Kate has shown signs of being delusional or paranoid. Somewhat shocked, I am aware of the debilitating effect her illness is having on her judgement as she reveals her inability to interpret her world in a realistic way. I do not contradict her, and I refrain from launching into what might ordinarily be an explanation about the workings of the human body. I simply listen, and commiserate.

For Kate has, in fact, become incontinent, and is no longer able to control her bladder or her bowel. It strikes me that this loss of capacity must be a crushing blow for someone as fastidious, as meticulous, as Kate Jowell has always been. But it is difficult to know how much of her current predicament she fathoms. At Carlucci's, Kate shows that she has, at least, an inkling that she has reached the point of no return. And it clearly torments her. 'No one understands,' she says, her eyes brimming with tears. I stroke her hand gently. 'I feel like a pariah,' she concludes.

Delusions – the mistaken belief in phenomena that have no factual existence – are common among those with Alzheimer's, occurring in up to 75 per cent of sufferers.

'They are simply mistaken beliefs, or judgments that are not reasonable,' explain Molloy and Caldwell.[198] The isolation that an Alzheimer's patient experiences is terrifying: a person with a delusion clings on to a belief with no reasonable evidence to the contrary. Others can see how inappropriate the belief is, but the person remains firmly convinced. 'In spite of profound memory loss, delusions are often held over long periods of time.'[199]

The anguish Kate shows is not new. Lately, her daily ablutions have become nightmarish – for her, and also for her caregivers. She is no longer able to take a shower on her own, having scalded herself just a few days before by turning on the hot-water tap and then forgetting how to turn it off. So she bathes instead, with Eunice's help, and this loss of privacy, of the ability to perform an ordinary daily cleansing ritual on her own, is deeply disturbing – a feeling that is clearly compounded by her incapacity to voice her feelings of frustration and despair.

The sequential action demanded by certain activities bewilders her – there are too many steps to follow – and as a result Kate has become, on rare occasions, uncooperative. Her once-groomed appearance is also slipping. She resists having her hair washed; she no longer wears her signature red lipstick.

We have had our usual cup of coffee, and as we make our way back to Glencoe Road, Kate's distress deepens. At the front door, with its wayward, welcoming palm, she bursts into tears and sobs uncontrollably. I hold her close, murmuring words of comfort. I am not sure how to lessen her pain, her confusion. She recovers, with some embarrassment. 'You are the only one who listens to me; you are so civilised,' she tells me. Her words touch me deeply, but they are no less bewildering for this. After all, if I am the only one who listens, what is it she believes I am hearing?

part four

COMMANDING
ATTENTION

10

In Her Own Voice

(1980)

HER CAREER HAD had many highlights, but Kate Jowell came fully into her own in 1980. After seven years at the Business School, she was appointed assistant director. But the competitive environment brought its own set of problems: Kate's rapid rise in business academia attracted the animosity of some of her male colleagues. John Simpson, director of the Business School at the time, recalls that it 'took a long time' for her colleagues to accept her.[200] He puts it down, in part, to 'chauvinism'. But her colleagues' main bone of contention was Kate's relative inexperience, and the fact that she initially did not have a clear-cut area of expertise.

Simpson, during his tenure as director (from 1979 to 1986), had appointed lecturers who were recognised experts in their fields. Some were not academics as such, but all were highly qualified, with doctorates in appropriate areas of expertise. Kate Jowell lacked this academic status. 'She was working on a doctoral thesis on black trade unionism at the time, but it was far from finished, and she did not have many academic articles to her name,' Simpson explains. Certain lecturers had a problem with this, which, Simpson believes, was 'understandable'.

Kate did not allow this barbed reaction to her success to affect her. She responded with her usual cool reserve, which was possibly interpreted as haughty arrogance. Yet, as one not given to passionate public displays, this was simply her way of coping. As Simpson observes, 'She just moved away from the animosity.' This would not have been easy, but Kate Jowell was an 'incredibly tenacious' woman. 'Once she set her sights on something, she just never let it go. She had her own vision, too, and she was ambitious, which was fine, but the other Business School lecturers would not let her forget that they were highly qualified, and highly regarded by the academic community, and she was not,' Simpson notes.[201]

But her increasing stature outside the stuffy academic world more than compensated for this. She continued to gain recognition in the labour field. In March 1980, in a *Sunday Times* article, she was described as a 'leading authority on black–white industrial relations'.[202] This widely read national newspaper was reporting on a speech Kate had delivered – on the state of industrial relations in South Africa – to the newly formed Cape Society of Chartered Accountants.

Engaging with her audience, she said that while the subject of industrial relations might not normally interest chartered accountants, there were good reasons why it should: 'We all like to live stable and comfortable lives with the minimum of stress – we expect the garbage to be collected, the post to be delivered and the banks to be open for business,' she began.[203] She went on to argue that chartered accountants are a significant pressure group in society, and it was important for them to understand South Africa's industrial relations climate so that they could make an informed contribution to pressure for change in legislation or social attitudes.

Kate predicted, as she had done in the past, that in the years to come, management's attitude to growing trade union power would be crucial to industrial peace. While South Africa had a relatively peaceful industrial climate compared with Britain's 'dismal record of industrial unrest', she cautioned that there was enormous potential for conflict in South Africa. 'Our environment is immensely more conflict-prone, though the issue is not whether conflict can be avoided, but whether the mechanisms we have in this country for channelling that conflict – with the least disruption – will stand up to the immense new pressures being put on them,' she contended.[204]

Characteristically, she presented a balanced argument, saying that while it would be important for black trade unions to 'put themselves within the constraints of legislation covering industrial relations', it would be equally important for management to 'discard the all-too-prevalent "tell-them-to-go-to-hell" attitude towards groups of workers'. Kate's political savvy was clear: 'One cannot deny the legacy of history. It is an unfortunate fact that because we have excluded blacks from legitimate trade union membership for so long, we have emphasised their political status rather than their status as workers.'

Strikes by black workers were therefore regarded as politically motivated and a threat to national security, and this had led to a more 'rapid politicisation of unions and workers'.[205] Kate elaborated: 'If the word "political" is used to describe the wish to redress disadvantages, to close the wage gap and press for opening of equal opportunities, there is no doubt that black trade unions will be used politically. If, of course, by "political" one means the wish to use trade unions to bring about the destruction of a political system and its replacement with another … all I can say is that there are many other avenues open to people for this kind of subversion of the status quo, even in our highly regimented society.'[206]

Kate saw a danger in union movements being used for political ends, but put her hopes in the constraining influence of the law and 'a system of bargaining and institutional arrangements that are visible and above board'.[207]

Kate spoke her mind, and the insight she brought to her subject is evident in the logic of her arguments. She continued to air her liberal views with confidence, even though she was now a member of the influential National Manpower Commission. By not toeing the ruling National Party's line, she could easily have scuppered her career opportunities. While her own political instincts were clearly liberal, her greatest strength was her ability to detach herself from the situation and assess the dynamics of change. Albie Sachs's prescient observation – that Kate was not 'stricken by the mores of white upper-middle-class southern African ladyship' – attests to this.[208]

Even though she was an establishment figure, Kate was able to articulate her alternative vision. This was because she had the capacity to imagine, and feel comfortable with, something other than the status quo, the normal world of white South Africans – a 'normality' that constrained their conceptions of what was possible or desirable. 'We must all ensure that by our actions within our companies and within the national forums open to us that we create the kind of society that the majority of people will want to preserve,' she concluded in her address to the chartered accountants' association.[209]

In June 1980 she was openly critical of the government's intervention to end a three-month strike in Cape Town by 800 meat-industry workers. The workers' defeat 'was not a victory for anyone', she noted. 'If the parties had come to some kind of agreement, then at least we would know that something had been learnt about the art of negotiation and compromise – rather than the damaging game of who wields the biggest stick.'[210]

Kate warned that confrontation had no value in industrial relations, not even in the short term. It gave the authorities an excuse for gate-crashing what should be a private party between unions and managers. A natural mediator, Kate believed that the only way to resolve disputes was by the time-honoured means of collective bargaining. Unions and managers 'should not look to outside intervention,' she said, 'whether it's in the form of police action or consumer boycotts or whatever.'[211]

Kate's public profile continued to grow, and she handled this with ease and confidence, bringing clarity and wisdom to national debates. She baulked at any suggestion that her prominence was partly due to her being an authoritative woman in a man's world, and embraced each challenge and opportunity that came her way.

Her commitment impressed, yet confounded, people. 'I always had great difficulty understanding why Kate was willing to put such effort into all these things,' says Naas Steenkamp, a fellow member of the National Manpower Commission and an influential executive in the mining industry, now retired, 'for she was not a social activist.'[212]

Steenkamp was especially struck by her professional directness. 'She was always someone with a straightforward agenda, and that was so evident within the Manpower Commission where, in a couple of weeks, she had everyone eating out of the palm of her hand.' Even the grey-shoed civil servants regarded Kate with 'awe'. Yet she didn't resort to what Steenkamp calls 'feminine wiles': 'She was matter-of-fact, always modest, never personal.' Even so, Kate's striking femininity did not go unnoticed. Steenkamp recalls an occasion when she walked into the Manpower Commission's meeting room in the Laboria Building in Pretoria. The morning sun was streaming into the room as she came through the door-way, casting her slim figure into sharp silhouette. 'She was wearing a yellow dress and looked gorgeous, but she was unaware of her impact,' he recalls. And unaffected by it, too. For when Steenkamp later told her about the incident, she was 'strangely indifferent to it'.

Steenkamp, a law graduate who entered the Foreign Service in 1959 and worked in London as third secretary – with a stint as private secretary to the High Commissioner – later entered the world of business. He ended up as executive director of Gencor (which was absorbed into Billiton, later to merge with BHP to become BHP Billiton, one of the largest mining houses in the world). Dapper and urbane, Steenkamp brought to his role in business the tact of a diplomat and a visionary professionalism that helped erode the intransigence and rigidity that dogged Gencor's labour relations. Because of his effectiveness, he became the group's representative at the Chamber of Mines, twice serving as its president.

Given Kate's prominence in the labour arena, it was only a matter of time before their paths would cross in the late 1970s. Steenkamp was chairman of the Industrial Relations Committee of the Wiehahn Com-mission at the time. In examining the broad issue of discrimination, it was inevitable that the commission also decided to consider discrimination on the grounds of gender. 'So we established a sub-committee to look into it, and cast about for someone with the right credentials … that's when Kate came into my life. She led the action of her own accord.'

Steenkamp took an immediate liking to Kate. She was thorough, and even when she differed with committee members, she was adroit at handling what Steenkamp calls the 'innate tensions' that arose from the fact that all fourteen commissioners were men. One of the proposals adopted by the Wiehahn Commission was the creation of a National Manpower Commission to spearhead South Africa's labour reforms. Kate and Naas Steenkamp would go on to be key members of the commission, facilitating change and, ultimately, labour legislation that would alter the course of South African history.

As Steenkamp notes, it was a rare and unique opportunity for two individuals outside the realm of politics to contribute to shaping national policy. Kate had a significant impact, which was all the more remarkable given the fact that the working language of the Manpower Commission, and the labour ministry, was Afrikaans – a language foreign to a former Rhodesian national.

'Kate had to do her work for the commission with a dictionary by her side,' Steenkamp recalls. 'It was phenomenal that she could conduct an informed debate on a subject with which she'd familiarised herself in a language she didn't really understand.' When she felt completely at sea, she'd call Steenkamp aside and ask for fifteen minutes of his time so that she could be sure her grasp of matters was accurate and sound.

Her dedication impressed Steenkamp: 'She really was a very hard worker, and one of the reasons for her efficiency was this Protestant work ethic.' Even though Kate lived in Cape Town, she'd fly to Pretoria for 'the most insignificant meetings', Steenkamp remembers. 'She'd arrive at the Laboria Building and make a direct contribution to proposals that would ultimately become recommendations of the commission. Her talent for analysis was critical to her performance. She was not a radical innovator, but always very well-informed and balanced in her thinking.'[213] These qualities were much in evidence, so Kate's opinions were valued and sought-after.

South Africa was entering a decade of rapid and radical change, and she was approached by the *Weekend Argus* in July of 1980 to comment on Prime Minister PW Botha's announcement that his government had accepted in principle the separate taxation of married women. Her viewpoint was that this could be 'incredibly beneficial' and might serve to lure professional and other highly qualified women back to the workplace.[214] It would be 'very good news indeed' if the government accepted that the contribution made by women was not marginal.

However, Kate's enthusiasm was tempered by her suspicion of a government that was slow to change, for it had previously shown reluctance to tax married women separately. 'I'm not sanguine about this,' she told *Weekend Argus.* 'A while ago the Brown Report concluded that separate taxation was equitable, and this is at odds with the apparent new view by the government and its tax experts.'[215]

Still, she believed there were several ways of introducing separate taxation without weakening the position of women in certain income brackets. If women were taxed separately, she concluded, 'all of us would be so much better off.'[216]

Shortly after the newspaper report was published, Kate went on a six-month sabbatical. She spent four months in the United States, in Boston, as a visiting fellow of the Sloan School of Management at the Massachusetts Institute of Technology (MIT). While there, she undertook research for her doctoral thesis, and also for the National Manpower Commission.

Her children were too young to be separated from their mother, so Kate took them – and their nanny – with her to Boston. Neil remained in Cape Town, visiting his wife and daughters on two occasions while they were living in the United States.

'Kate left Cape Town in the middle of the South African summer,' Neil recalls. 'I remember the season because when I arrived in Boston I tried to do some cycling, but the cycling tours had already ended.'[217]

In Boston, Kate ran into her former student Harris Gordon, and his wife, photographer Tessa Frootko Gordon, who had immigrated to the United States for political reasons. Harris remembers Kate as being 'slender, attractive, fairly wispy'. He is vague about how they learnt she was living in Boston. 'I must have attended one of her lectures at MIT … I am not really sure how we connected. But I invited her to supper one evening, and she came alone. It was a very cold night, the eve of an American public holiday,' he says. 'Tessa and I were new to the country, and we were struggling, and we threw together a simple supper, serving her canned soup, or something. She may have expected something else, but she was very gracious, and quite a lady.'[218]

At the time, South Africa was the pariah of the Western world. Harris notes that it was 'very rare for a South African to show up in the States'. One South African who was expected to put in an appearance, though – to deliver a lecture at MIT – was Percy Qoboza, former editor of *City Press*. Qoboza had been invited to speak at MIT by Robert (Bob) Rotberg, professor of political science and history, a position he held for twenty years. Rotberg is an esteemed academic and influential author, and has been an observer of the American political scene for more than forty years. He had a special interest in South Africa – hence the invitation to Qoboza.

Kate and Neil were curious to hear what Qoboza might have to say, but, according to Neil, 'he didn't show up'. There were about seventy people in the lecture theatre. Kate and Neil were sitting close to the front of the auditorium, in the third row. After waiting for about fifteen minutes, Rotberg stood up and announced that the guest speaker had failed to arrive.

'Bob, as he is known to friends, initiated a discussion on South Africa, on an aspect that was not Kate's field of speciality,' Neil says. But she listened intently, and quickly realised that participating members of the audience were uninformed about South Africa. Unable to contain herself, she stood up and calmly presented a balanced alternative view. 'Bob was very impressed by her,' according to Neil. It was the start of a connection that lasted for decades.

Bob Rotberg now lectures at Harvard University, where he directs the Program on Intrastate Conflict and Conflict Resolution at the Kennedy School of Government. His particular interest has always been contemporary American policy. A regular visitor to South Africa, he was, for professional as well as personal reasons, in Johannesburg when I tracked him down to talk about Kate Jowell. 'My first impressions of her, and they have remained unaltered through the years, were of a lively, bright and interesting person,' he begins.[219] He has known her for twenty-three years and says that, as friendships go, he and Kate were always more than casual acquaintances, though never very close.

'We didn't get to the revealing parts of friendship. She is not that way inclined, and neither am I. She always kept her personal life to herself. What I knew about her private life I knew by inference, or things other people had told me.'

Bob's visits to Cape Town have declined somewhat over the years, but in the early 1980s he was a regular dinner-party guest – and often a house guest, too – at both Jowell homes. The dinner parties, he says, were 'in the grand style, with lots of guests. There was the usual friendly chatting, with all sorts of interesting people present. I was usually more to the left of anyone else in the room, certainly during the apartheid years,' he notes.

Amid the cards in Kate's little navy box, where she recorded personal details of her dinner parties and her guests, there is a separate card for Bob and Joanna Rotberg. The first entry is in 1981, the last in 1996. Kate noted that Joanna 'drinks rooibos tea', though she seemed in doubt as to their preference for pudding. Another long-standing friend of the Jowells – Virginia Ogilvie Thompson – was also a mutual friend of the Rotbergs. Her name, abbreviated to VOT, appears often on Kate's cards.

At one dinner party, on 31 January 1986, Kate and Neil entertained Virginia, the Rotbergs, Meyer Feldberg, Joop de Loor – director-general of finance at the time – and Dawid de Villiers. Kate served an elegant meal: snoek soufflé, chicken Elizabeth, ginger melon with ginger ice. The wine was Chardonnay. 'Not sure if D de V likes him,' Kate noted enigmatically, her discretion coming into play even in her private papers.

Kate's 1980 sabbatical was productive. But it was not without its challenges: she was on her own in a foreign country, with two small children to look after, and a demanding work schedule. Often, the bitterly cold American winter was not on her side. On some mornings she would head outside, only to be confronted with a car that was shrouded in snow. 'I remember her telling us how her nanny had to help her dig the car out,' says Tessa Frootko Gordon. But the year ended in triumph when Kate became the first – and only – woman appointed, for a three-year period, to the Standing Commission of Inquiry into the Taxation Policy of the Republic of South Africa. Her appointment coincided with that of Dr Simon Brand, economic adviser to the prime minister, HV Hefer, a Johannesburg accountant, and businessman Derek Keys, chairman of the National Discount House.

Kate's appointment to the commission was generally well received, and especially lauded in several circles. It was also widely reported in the national press: 'A woman's voice on taxation', the Durban-based *Daily News* announced; 'Government appoints woman to taxing commission', read the headline of an article that appeared in Johannesburg's daily, *The Star*; 'UCT woman named for tax commission', the Cape Town afternoon paper, *The Argus*, noted; and 'At last we have a voice! A woman in the world of finance … Appointment hailed as breakthrough,' the *Weekend Argus* heralded.

Kate was in her element. 'Naturally I am pleased that I have been asked to serve on the commission,' she told Gorry Bowes Taylor in a telephone interview from New York. 'Tax programmes largely reflect a government's industrial and social policies, and I feel privileged to have been given a chance to take part in our continuing debate.'[220]

Professional women were impressed by her appointment. They saw it as a breakthrough, an opportunity for women's needs and concerns to be heard and addressed. It was also a sign that working women were being recognised – by the government and by society – as important role-players in the South African economy.[221] In an effusive report, journalist Sue Garbett wrote: 'Kate Jowell is a brilliant woman whose brilliant career has been given a further shine by her appointment to the Standing Commission of Inquiry into the Taxation Policy of the Republic.'[222]

Other women who voiced their approval of Kate's appointment were luminaries like Progressive Party Member of Parliament Helen Suzman, and consumer expert and President's Council member Margaret Lessing.

'This is an excellent appointment,' Helen Suzman is quoted as saying. 'I have no doubt Mrs Jowell will pay special attention to the thorny problem of separate taxation for married working women.'[223] Suzman felt that Kate's inclusion in the commission line-up was 'certainly an improvement on the previously chauvinistic attitude of the government'.

Adèle van der Spuy, who had lobbied for a system of separate taxation for married women for six years and led a delegation to convince Prime Minister PW Botha of their case, said Kate's appointment to the commission was 'absolutely tremendous'. She elaborated: 'Never before in the history of this country have women had a voice in finance. We can now hope for positive tax results as well as equal pay for men and women in the teaching profession.'

Christiane Duval, who was at this stage an adviser to the Johannesburg Chamber of Commerce, was pleased about Kate's new role. Kate's appointment was 'a breakthrough', Duval conceded, even though she felt that the government would not have made it 'without suggestions from us women. At last we feel the Department of Finance is taking a serious look at women.'[224]

Once again, Kate found herself pigeonholed into representing women's interests. She handled the situation with her usual tact, saying that while the taxation of married women would probably be on the commission's agenda 'if only because of the current argument about whether or not it keeps skilled women from working', there were other pressing issues to be considered. She pointed out that the taxation of married women was by no means the most important one South Africa faced on the tax front. Other issues – for example the role tax policy might play in alleviating the unemployment rate – were more critical in addressing economic development.[225]

No doubt frustrated at being perceived yet again as a 'token woman', Kate reiterated that she did not approve of 'this kind of stereotyping'. However, she accepted that, as she was the only female member of the commission, women would expect her to present their case. She expressed the hope that she would do so 'competently and fairly'.[226]

The year was drawing to a close. Kate was triumphant. Then, to top it all, in November 1980, she was one of twenty-two nominees for *The Star*'s Woman of the Year Award. One of only two Capetonians nominated – the other was human rights lobbyist Professor Erika Theron – Kate was in good company. The nominees included achievers in a variety of fields – actresses Nomsa Nene and Sandra Prinsloo, dean of the University of the Witwatersrand Law School Professor Louise Tager, as well as Dr Rookaya Docrat Moolla, superintendent of Stanger Provincial Hospital in Natal, and Sarah Dombo, the first woman branch manager of the Permanent Life Assurance Company. Kate didn't win the award, but her nomination, at the age of forty, was more than gratifying.

~

June 2003. By now, I have known Kate Jowell for six months. It has been a rewarding yet bewildering time, for me as much as for her, I suspect. I am attempting to piece together her life story, to find her voice – without her being able to speak for herself. There are so many things I want, and need, to ask her. But there can be no answers. I can, therefore, enter the mind of the astute, clear-headed thinker I am writing about only by imagining what she might have said. My task is all the more difficult because we have no shared history; unlike that of biographer AN Wilson, whose friendship with his subject, Iris Murdoch, spanned thirty years. And yet, even Wilson admits that his biography, *Iris Murdoch – As I Knew Her*, is nothing more than 'an attempt to get hold of IM, to prise out her secret, as one might use a pin to take a winkle from its shell'.[227]

My task seems even more daunting. And yet, prising out Kate's secrets, attempting to reveal the essence of who she was and the way she engaged with her world, has been an enlightening process. We have, between us, developed a pattern of communicating. Instead of bombarding her with questions that inevitably begin with the words, 'Do you remember …?' – words she probably dreads – I have tried to put things to her in a way that may be less confrontational, less demanding. I have often read to her – not only the transcripts of my interviews with former colleagues, friends, acquaintances, her children, her husband, her brother, but also things she has written, or the rough drafts of our project, her memoir.

I have become her contact with the outside world, carrying greetings to her from people who were once her colleagues, a vital part of life as she once knew it. She is able to piece together some things, respond to and expand on others. Increasingly, though, she is simply at a loss for words, and I sometimes struggle to understand whether she truly has, in a given moment, no recollection of a person or an event, or whether she is simply not able to articulate her thoughts, to put them into words, to speak her mind. It is at times like this that I am most aware of the effect of Alzheimer's. It is so blatant, and so irrevocable.

Increasingly, Neil is experiencing this too. During one of our chats at his Trencor office, he says that most people have the misguided view that Alzheimer's damages the sufferer's memory only. 'Very few people understand how it really impacts on, and erodes, one's daily life,' he soberly states.[228] Kate's delusions have been unsettling, and upsetting, to say the least. When he is at home to witness the symptoms, he deals with the situation pragmatically. 'You don't find it troubling at the time, when you're dealing with it, but on reflection, it hits you.'

In January 2003, Kate's neurologist, Dr John Gardiner, had warned Neil: 'The Kate you know will be gone in six months' time.' This time has now arrived. Reflecting on this, Neil is overcome with emotion. Roughly, with the palms of his hands, he wipes tears from his eyes. 'For a long time she had been stable, but suddenly I can see a very clear destruction of her personality. Also, she could always see the funny side of things, but she is now losing her sense of humour too.'

He is right. Kate's delusions, and the medication she is now taking to counteract their destabilising effect, have not only subdued her, but robbed her of her spark, her wit. These are cruel reminders that 'Mr Alzheimer's' is relentlessly at work.

Neil also points out that his relationship with his wife, and their domestic routine, have changed profoundly. 'I obviously can't communicate with her like I used to. We never used to watch much TV, but we've watched a fair bit in the past three years. I got satellite television so that Kate would be occupied during the day. She likes to watch certain BBC programmes – *Hard Talk* and *BBC News* – and we watch those at night, and it takes up most of our evenings.'[229]

After he has helped Kate to bed, usually at about 9.30 p.m., he turns his attention to work matters, communicating with colleagues in the United States. 'I have coped with Kate's illness by keeping busy,' he says.

~

Alzheimer's is usually impossible to diagnose until after the patient is dead. The formal diagnosis of most sufferers of the disease is, therefore, 'probable Alzheimer's disease'. David Shenk explains: 'A definitive determination requires evidence of both plaques and tangles – which cannot be obtained without drilling into the patient's skull, snipping a tiny piece of brain tissue and examining it under a microscope.'[230] But brain biopsies are invasive procedures, and are generally not performed on patients whose lives are not immediately threatened.

One of the defining characteristics of Alzheimer's – and a key way of distinguishing it from other types of dementia – is its stealth. It is not an abrupt disease. Slowly, almost imperceptibly, it sets in, and then drifts from one stage to the next in what Shenk aptly terms 'a slow-motion haze'.

'Creeping diseases blur the boundaries in such a way that they can undermine our basic assumptions of illness.'[231]

Today, a diagnosis of 'probable Alzheimer's' can be made through a number of tests that usually start with a simple quiz: What is today's date? What day of the week is it? What city do we live in? And so on. Patients are also asked to count backwards, to repeat the names of objects that have just been mentioned to them, to fold a piece of paper, to write a sentence, to draw a circle, a triangle, a rectangle. This 'neurological obstacle course' is called the Mini Mental State Examination (MMSE), and was introduced worldwide in 1975 as a crude but effective way of detecting problems patients experience with time and place orientation, object registration, abstract thinking, recall, and verbal and written cognition. A person with 'normal' functioning will score very close to the perfect 30 points in an MMSE, while a person with early-to-moderate dementia will generally fall below 24.[232]

Kate first started doing Mini Mentals and another test – the slightly more elaborate Adas-COG test – in the latter half of 1999. Her test results, and the drug trials in which she has taken part, have been monitored by Alexandra Aleksic, a pharmacist who works with Dr John Gardiner. Explaining how the Mini Mentals are conducted, Aleksic says of patients being put through a series of tests: 'Some of them focus on the ability to recall words. For example, I show the patient three cards, depicting a dog, a mountain and a river. I ask her to tell me what she sees, then I put the cards down and test her ability to recall any of the images.'[233]

Aleksic says that Kate's vocabulary and her ability to recall the words she wants to use are unusually good for an Alzheimer's patient. 'She is very good with words, which is strange.' Kate still knows that she has five fingers on each hand. She can point up and down. But sometimes she battles to make a fist with her hand. She can no longer write, or draw. 'When I ask her to write "It's a lovely day today", she can write one or two letters, then she presents this to me as a complete sentence,' Aleksic explains.

Kate can draw a circle, but not a diamond shape or two overlapping rectangles. 'She knows her name, but the daily information that regulates our lives, like telling the time and today's date … she has no idea.'

Mini Mentals are similar to the Adas-COG tests, but Aleksic explains that they are not as complicated and include more questions involving arithmetic. 'I am always interested to see how Kate copes with the maths, because she has a degree in mathematics, but I have been shocked by her inability to do the simplest of sums.'

She can also see a marked change in the way Kate walks. 'When she first started coming for the tests, she'd stride into our rooms. She'd have the newspapers under her arm, and she'd flip through them. Now she shuffles … this is when the reality of Alzheimer's really hits you. To see such a capable woman struck down in her prime. Even though she still seems interested in things, I can see a huge deterioration since she was here two months ago,' Aleksic says.[234]

All this is true, and as a result Kate's days are increasingly long and lonely. Her seclusion is so much more pronounced now than when I first met her. Friends visit her less and less frequently. They are depressed and devastated by the change in her – frightened, no doubt, by her condition.

Nowadays, Kate's only forays into the outside world are her Wednesday-morning drives, her outings with Neil and our visits to Carlucci's. Occasionally I take her somewhere else, but the routine of a familiar environment makes her feel secure. Recently, on returning home after our usual stint at Carlucci's, she confided, 'Sometimes I am scared here on my own.'

No longer a haven, the Glencoe Road house has become a hostile place. Kate observes that she feels her worst 'on the weekend, when Neil goes out'. I suggest she calls Justine when she's feeling anxious – but typically, not wanting to intrude on her daughter's busy life, Kate spurns the idea. Shaking her head, she replies, 'I don't like to disturb Justine.'

'Well, then, you must call me,' I offer. She smiles wistfully, but doesn't answer. In that instant I know that she will not call.

It is only when I take leave of her, when I drive away, that I realise that even if she were willing to reach out, to ask for help, the simple act of using a telephone is now beyond her capability. Finding the telephone number, deciphering the numerals, punching them into the phone … this everyday act of communication, of staying in touch, of making oneself heard, is completely beyond her reach.

I am also struck by the realisation of Kate's continuing courage and humour in the face of all this. Just today, as we returned from Carlucci's, as she tentatively negotiated her way down the steep staircase at the entrance to the house, she cheerily greeted Eunice with the words, 'I'm back, Eunice … like a bad penny!' Then her clear, ringing laughter echoed through the large reception area.

I can still hear it as I drive away.

II

Distinguished Woman

(1981–83)

K ATE RETURNED HOME from her United States sojourn at the
end of 1980 to a country facing internal unrest, hostile front-line
states, economic depression and a broadening international pro-sanctions
campaign. Prime Minister PW Botha, who had come to power in 1978,
increasingly warned those clamouring for political change that, as long
as he was in charge, 'one person, one vote' was out of the question.

But his messages were often contradictory. For it was Botha who
coined the phrase 'adapt or die', which would later become a rallying cry
for reform. Addressing white South Africans who opposed change, he
cautioned, 'The world does not remain the same, and if we as government
want to act in the best interests of the country in a changing world, then
we have to be prepared to adapt our policy to those things that make
adjustment necessary. Otherwise we die.'

However, like his predecessors Hendrik Verwoerd and John Vorster,
Botha was determined to preserve the status quo, to keep political power
in white hands. 'In order to maintain that power, he was prepared to
make a trade-off: a relaxation of laws governing social and economic
apartheid in return for continued white control of the Republic.' [235]

In her role as a labour commentator and, increasingly, an industrial
relations consultant, Kate was quick to analyse the government's game
plan. In 1981, speaking at the annual dinner of the Cape of Good Hope

Soroptimists, she said the changes in South Africa's labour laws had 'put a nail in the coffin of civilised labour policy', one of the cornerstones of apartheid.[236] And when a cornerstone of a building was removed, she pointed out, the whole edifice was likely to fall over.

However, even though the government had combed its legislation 'to tidy it up' and rewritten 'every clause relating to job opportunities or wages ... to exclude discrimination on the basis of race or sex or colour', this was, basically, a pointless exercise until radical political change came about. Kate put the question to her audience: 'Can we embrace, as we have now done, the principle that merit and ability will be the only criteria for a man's role in the economy without bringing about a change in a wide political sphere?'

She went on to express her own firm viewpoint: 'I think not. We cannot give blacks equal access to work opportunities without them developing power and economic muscle to dictate the conditions under which they would like to operate in the workplace.' Kate warned that a lack of political and economic opportunity would lead to a situation where organised labour would demand the kind of political change that would enable such a scenario to come into being.[237]

Kate went on to contend that it was impossible to implement a policy of equal opportunity based on merit and ability unless those involved had 'equal opportunities to develop to a level where they, in fact, have merit and ability'. As long as there were policies of segregated education, which inevitably meant 'differential standards of education', segregated housing, which meant 'inferior housing for some', and segregated areas where people might live, there would be inferior facilities for certain groups of people. In such a social and political environment, it could not be argued convincingly that people had equal opportunities. Kate pointed out the simple reality that managers had long since discovered: 'A BComm degree from Turfloop isn't remotely the same as a BComm from UCT.'

If the government failed to implement the broader social changes that were needed, the pressure for change would be focused exclusively on the workplace. Kate saw that the consequence would be political tension and disruptive strike action. 'No rational government can endure economic dislocation,' she said, going on to state with her usual frankness: 'To many black minds, apartheid and free enterprise must seem to be synonymous. How far we can detach the two will depend on how soon and how quickly we move on to a more just society ... to retain the best of the society that we have while dispensing with the unjust, I think we have to make capitalism acceptable and dissolve the granite face of apartheid.'[238] She conceded, however, that this would require a massive attempt by everyone concerned to promote positive change.

Kate's ability to analyse and interpret the political situation in a fiercely independent way – and to offer considered solutions to complex problems – ensured that her services were much in demand. Neil Jowell recalls her being approached by construction giant Murray & Roberts to assist with pressing labour issues. 'The chairman told her that they were not utilising their people to their full potential, and they wanted her to do a survey on how they could remedy the situation.'[239] It was, as Neil points out, a significant job for someone as young as Kate was at the time. But she was confident of her abilities and took up the challenge, visiting the company's main sites in Cape Town, Durban and Johannesburg.

Ironically, though, Murray & Roberts handled her visit insensitively, providing her with a fine example of a short-sighted approach to the management of people. Neil tells the story with a glint in his eye: 'They took her to three clubs, including the Rand Club in Johannesburg and the Durban Club, which admitted only male members.' As a woman, Kate had to enter the Durban Club via the back door! Perhaps the company was acknowledging, albeit in a strange way, that they had accepted her into their inner circle, that she was 'one of the boys'.

But Kate would certainly not have seen it that way. She had never defined herself, or her abilities, in terms of her gender. She had never set out to be 'one of the boys'. Her simple goal was to use her talents and skills to the best of her ability. If this meant encroaching on male territory, she had the guts, and the intellect, to pull it off. She would therefore have found the lunch neither an amusing nor a heartening experience.

Taking up the story, Neil describes Kate's dinner with the company's top executives at the Rand Club, which had reciprocity with the Durban Club. He observes rather wryly that in Cape Town the company hosted her at Kelvin Grove, which for many years did not admit Jewish members.

'I don't think Murray & Roberts realised their actions were discriminatory until Kate pointed it out to them when she delivered her final report on how the company could use its people to greater effect,' Neil muses. 'She made the point that we go about our business without noticing the inherent discrimination in things we do on a daily basis.'[240]

But, to the company's credit, they were so impressed by her observations and advice that she was mentioned by name in the annual *Chairman's Report* by Des Baker, who was, at the time, chairman of Murray & Roberts. 'It was unheard of to mention a consultant's name in an annual report, and I have rarely seen it since,' Neil explains with more than a hint of pride.[241]

~

At the University of Cape Town Graduate School of Business, Kate continued to gain credibility. But the doctoral thesis she'd begun was starting to lose its appeal. Neil explains that while she did, in fact, spend 'a fair bit of time on it', she got side-tracked. 'She didn't really want to spend two years on a specific field, working on a doctorate. She preferred the business of diversity,' Neil says.[242]

Perhaps it was simply a case of not having enough time. Kate Jowell was an extraordinarily busy woman, fulfilling not only her commitments to her husband and her two small children, but also her taxing lecturing duties at the Business School, and on top of this she was a member of the National Manpower Commission and of the Standing Commission of Inquiry into the Taxation Policy of the Republic. It is perhaps no coincidence that, in a decade in which the term 'Superwoman' was coined, Kate's schedule represented an almost superhuman list of duties.

To top it all, she was at the time in great demand as a labour consultant, flying around South Africa to advise companies – from the giant mining houses to smaller concerns – on how to resolve workplace strife and improve productivity. And so, the unfinished doctorate on black trade unionism remains perhaps the only loose end in her ordered life. For Kate Jowell was not the kind of person to abandon a project, to throw in the towel.

The fact that Kate was under a lot of pressure at the time was clear to her supervisor, Dr James Leatt.[243] She was, essentially, attempting a PhD in a discipline in which she lacked a solid academic background. So, she'd had to start from scratch, reading all the relevant literature, going back to basic economics before moving, for example, to related political issues. According to John Simpson, all this probably proved too time-consuming, and it's likely that Kate abandoned the exercise because she felt that she didn't need a doctorate.

The situation is very different today, says Simpson, since without a PhD a lecturer is highly unlikely to be promoted to a senior position. Because Kate was working in a new field, however, she soon developed a reputation as an authority in that field, and in the light of this, Simpson's question is an interesting one: 'Did she really need a PhD? Well, she obviously made up her mind that she didn't.'[244]

From time to time I have asked Kate herself about this one part of her life, her career, which seems incomplete. It is a question she cannot answer. Often, with a perplexed look, she has replied, 'I don't know. I can't remember.' I take care not to put words in her mouth, to ask leading questions. I once said to her, 'Did you feel it was unnecessary because you were so busy, and your career was taking off with or without your having a doctorate?' Her reply – which was, 'Yes, I think so' – left me feeling uncertain about whether or not she really meant this, or was simply at a loss for words.

What is certain, though, is that Kate concentrated her mind on developing new course material for her pioneering field. Industrial relations was not a study option at the Business School when Kate did her MBA in 1973. When she joined the Business School staff the following year, she took over the Manpower Development course and developed its Industrial Relations content until it was introduced as a core course of the Business School's MBA programme in 1980. This was a major challenge – and a major achievement – for Kate had no relevant source material, or case studies, to draw on.

In spite of drastic and fundamental changes to South Africa's labour scene at the time, it was widely acknowledged that tangible progress remained agonisingly slow.

Whatever revolution may have taken place existed 'more in the legal structure, in philosophy and in rhetoric than in action'. [245] The challenge, labour experts warned, had moved from the capacity of the government and business to permit change at all to whether they and the trade unions (both black and white) would move quickly enough to develop new partnerships. There were general misgivings that a failure to do so would result in an inability to exercise control over the course of change.

In one of her numerous media observations, Kate Jowell noted that legal recognition, legal assistance and the opportunity to bind employers to a legal agreement were essential to the survival of the black trade union movement. [246]

At the time, the Wiehahn Report estimated that between 55 000 and 70 000 workers – which, in 1977, constituted barely 1 per cent of the total black workforce of 7 million – were then believed to belong to twenty-seven black unregistered trade unions. But times were changing, and by June 1981 black membership of registered trade unions had increased to about 65 000, as compared with none in October 1979. This was in the wake of the Industrial Conciliation Amendment Act, which legalised black union membership.

Whenever and wherever she could, Kate emphasised the importance of political reform. In 1982, at a symposium organised by the Institute of Personnel Management, she spoke out for the need to close the wage gap and reduce the skill and opportunity gap, and the necessity of freeing blacks to compete on an equal footing in the workplace, 'without the shackles of influx control'. [247] Kate saw quite clearly that the forces of change were already happening outside the parameters of established political structures: 'The new trade unions themselves and some enlightened managers are moving us fast along the road to closing the wage and opportunity gaps.' She knew, however, that positive change needed to be managed, and that it therefore demanded a radical change throughout the entire political and social structure.

Kate was, however, sensitive to the deep anxieties of many of her fellow white citizens regarding the groundswell of change in the labour arena. Such fears were expressed by Conservative Party MP Frank le Roux, who warned Parliament that the Minister of Manpower would be remembered for scuppering the National Party's ship by saying 'goodbye, through his labour reforms, to the policy of separate development'.[248]

Kate refused to compromise, however, believing that the price to be paid for refusing political change would be far too high. Her career continued on an upward trajectory in 1981, attaining new heights – and reaping increasingly enthusiastic accolades. In August that year, she was one of seven women vying for the title of South Africa's Businesswoman of the Year. The other contenders were Pamela Levy, Margaret Lessing, Lucy Mvubelo, Velia Kirkpatrick, Johanna Schoeman and Sandra van der Merwe.

While Kate didn't win – the recipient of the award was Margaret Lessing – her nomination was yet again a reflection of her career status and her position as one of the country's top women. But that was not all. The following month, in September, Kate was appointed a member of the Western Cape board of Barclays National Bank.

As was the case with all her previous appointments, this was a significant one. Kate still had to contend with popular prejudice, however, and resisted the perception that she was a token woman. She fought hard to prove the legitimacy of her belief in equal rights and opportunities for women, and was an active voice in women's organisations.

It comes as no surprise, therefore, that she was present at the launch of the ground-breaking National Women's Bureau in 1981, the first official organisation in South Africa formed to represent the interests of working women. The launch of the Women's Bureau was something of a coup: women's groups had lobbied for its formation since 1964, but two successive prime ministers – Hendrik Verwoerd and John Vorster – had, for a collective period of seventeen years, refused their request for a national official body.

Margaret Lessing headed the newly formed organisation, and she attributed the government's change of attitude to the serious shortage of skilled employees at the time, and the fact that women were taking up their rightful place in the world of work and were therefore far more visible than before.[249]

Two years later, in 1983, Minister of Manpower Fanie Botha removed the long-standing ban on women working overtime and at night. The new legislation was well received, with Botha boldly declaring that the full gamut of women's organisations applauded the amendments. But he had not reckoned on Conservative Party Member of Parliament Bessie Scholtz, who claimed that the new law would further destabilise home life.

Once again, however, Kate Jowell saw the shape of the future, placing things in a historical context of rapid socio-political change: 'The new law is part of the embracing of the whole free enterprise ethic, which began in 1979 with the dismantling of some of the racially discriminatory laws in the labour field.'[250] She was referring, specifically, to the Wiehahn Commission, which had, inter alia, investigated the discriminatory restrictions facing working women.

Clearly, women's liberation was slow to arrive in South Africa. Clarifying the situation, Roberta Johnston, who headed the commission's Study Group on Women in Employment, explained that the removal of overtime restrictions was a priority: 'Women were deprived of working overtime to increase earnings, which went to men instead. We felt this was discriminatory.'[251] The reactionary position of the Conservative Party was ridiculed for its relegation of women to the lowly status of mere wives in the kitchen, and for ignoring the economic plight of single, divorced and widowed women.

While Kate was pleased with the government's amendments to a discriminatory employment law, she cautioned that legislation yet remained that was unsympathetic to women, curtailing the right of a pregnant woman to work, for example. Clearly, though, in the early 1980s, South Africa's working women were finding their collective voice and establishing themselves as a force with which to be reckoned.

Again, Kate Jowell was one of the front-runners.

~

July 2003. It is 10.30 a.m. and, unusually, Kate is running late. We are deviating today from our Carlucci's routine to watch a video at my home in Claremont. The recording is not a feature film, but a 1983 television debate on the taxation of married women, which was aired on the SABCTV actuality programme *Midweek*. The star of the show is Kate Jowell herself.

When Neil handed me the tape, he confessed that the video machine at Glencoe Road had been broken for some time. He had replaced it with a DVD player, which he bought soon after Kate took early retirement from the Business School. 'I thought she might like to watch movies while she was alone at home, that it would give her something to do,' he explains. I can't help wondering whether Kate has put the DVD player to much use at all, for since I met her in January, she has never once mentioned watching a DVD at home.

I am, yet again, struck by the irony of Kate's situation: this woman, who once engaged so keenly with a wide outside world, and who was once far too busy to go to the cinema, has now – when she has more than enough time on her hands – been robbed of the capacity to follow and enjoy the medium of film.

I am glumly pondering her fate, her isolation, her aloneness, when her elegant Audi pulls up outside. Her driver, Ivan Jacobus, who takes Kate for a weekly Wednesday-morning excursion, confesses that he had lost his way. Nonetheless, Kate is cheerful and happy to see me. We gingerly make our way along the slate pathway to my front door. She finds the dark tiles unsettling, and as her depth perception has been impaired by Alzheimer's, she seems to 'see' obstacles in the path and she tries to step over them. I convince her that the surface is even and, after navigating a short staircase, we are safely ensconced in the living room.

I seat her next to me, and she sits forward, on the edge of the couch. I press the TV remote-control's 'play' button and the strident *Midweek* tune heralds the start of the programme. It is called 'Till Tax Us Do Part'... In an instant, Kate and I are taken back twenty years, and we're listening to a heated debate on a pressing issue that concerned working women at the time: the double insult of being taxed jointly with their husbands, thereby not only losing their 'identity', but also having to pay more money to the Receiver of Revenue in the process.

The face of Norman Bisby beams at us from the screen. Introducing the programme, he states that more than 75 per cent of South Africa's married working women are dissatisfied with the tax system: 'The archetypal South African married woman is no longer merely a housewife, but a person who is playing an increasing role in the economy and is demanding rights as an independent individual.' His delivery is quick but oddly punctuated, and I glance at Kate to see if she is following what he is saying. Her face is inscrutable.

Panel chairman Nigel Murphy introduces the panellists, and quite suddenly Kate appears on the screen, looking somewhat severe. She is wearing a silky fern-green blouse that is at once feminine and demure, its collar – complete with bow detail – reaching her slim neck. Her short, glossy brown hair frames her face, but her large glasses – very much in vogue at the time – dwarf her delicate features and hide her lively eyes. Hers is a glamour with *gravitas*: her lips are coloured with her usual red lipstick, and while she is not power dressing on this occasion, her distinctly 1980s look, with its prim austerity, projects a serious intelligence. How different she seems here to the witty, self-effacing, light-hearted Kate I have grown fond of in recent months.

Her inclusion on the *Midweek* panel is in her capacity as a member of the Standing Commission of Inquiry into the Taxation Policy of the Republic. She is joined by two other women panellists: Sue Grant, women's editor of *The Star* newspaper, and Professor Carmen Nathan of the University of Bophuthatswana's School of Law. The male panellists are tax author Costa Divaris and Clive Kingon, tax structure development director of Inland Revenue.

The opening contributions from Carmen Nathan and Sue Grant underscore the dissatisfaction of women and the injustice of the tax system. Grant tells Nigel Murphy that, as a journalist, she has experienced huge reader reaction to the issue, the biggest reaction to any newspaper article she has written: 'There is extraordinary anger out there. I am not a tax expert, but I know what the person in the street feels like.'

I note with interest that Kate does not immediately side with the other women on the panel. She operates independently, and in her opening contribution to the debate sets out one of her key points: 'I think one has to distinguish between low-income and high-income couples. It's in the higher brackets that inequity is most felt, and I think the inequity is basically that the whole of the married woman's earnings are treated as incremental, as pin money on top of her husband's, and most married women do not want to be taxed incrementally, they want a full reward for a full effort. And that's where the inequity lies,' she concludes.

Other panellists make the point that the unfair tax system is keeping working women out of the job market at a time when South Africa sorely needs its skilled and professional workers. But Kingon points out that, in the seven years to 1983, the number of married women at work rose from 34 per cent to between 40 and 43 per cent. 'Tax is not keeping them away, but we have to look at what income categories they are in. Maybe a larger number going to work are those forced by economic circumstances to do so.'

Kate homes in on Kingon's point. 'Clive put his finger on it when he said one must distinguish between the number of women who are working and those who are working because they have a choice between work and leisure, or rather between two jobs and one job. People in the lower-income category have no choice, but those in the higher category may look at the incremental return and decide whether or not they want to go back to work.'

Her unique approach and the incontrovertible logic of her argument are impressive: 'High progressive marginal rates of tax exacerbate the problem, but this should not disguise the principle, which is the principle that deems a wife's salary to be her husband's, and lumping it on top of his as pin money to be taxed at his incremental rate.'

Costa Divaris underscores what he calls 'Kate's point' about the distinction between income groups by saying that 73 per cent of taxpayers in 1983 earned less than R12 000, and 'if you change the system, these people will end up paying more tax … they are the bulk of voters and they will not let you change the system'.

Kate refines the idea in the next series of exchanges. The word 'unfair' has been bandied about by the other panellists. Kate obviously feels it needs to be pinned down and qualified. So, partly in response to Nigel Murphy's efforts to steer the discussion towards defining ways to change the tax system and to decide if it is, in fact, desirable to do so, Kate responds: 'Well, it depends on how you change the system. There is any one of a number of options to change the system, but fairness is a political term because taxation is a form of social engineering all governments use to reorganise income distribution.'

Kate and I watch as we sit together on the couch, and I can't help wondering to what extent she is able to follow the intricacies of the argument today. Her silence, which contrasts starkly with the animated Kate on the screen, speaks volumes.

'Are you saying there is no way to achieve a more equitable system?' Murphy demands of her. 'No,' she calmly responds, 'there are plenty of ways, but there is no tax change that can be made that does not end up with someone being worse off than someone else, and the government decides who it wants to squeeze at any point for political reasons.'

I have watched this video recording several times now, and each time

I am more impressed by Kate Jowell's grasp of an argument, her ability to follow through and reach a well-reasoned conclusion without being deflected. Perhaps I find it particularly fascinating because this is a woman I know and yet do not know. The Kate who is sitting next to me, and who is now fidgeting, probably because she's lost the thread of the argument and is trying to hide her distress, is a different person from the cool, articulate woman on the screen. In-between playing with her sleeve, Kate watches her other self, this woman on the screen who is and is not her, but she says nothing. Occasionally, however, after she's made a point on screen, she will turn to me and say, with a somewhat inscrutable grin, 'That's my line.' For the rest of the time she is mute, merely wringing her hands.

On screen, Kate gestures eloquently, using her hands to great effect as she talks, emphasising her contention that the conflicting interests of various lobby groups are influential in shaping tax policy. 'The Directorate of Finance gets a certain amount of tax from different sources,' she says, 'and all of them are asking him to reduce their load. There is the married couples' lobby, the beer lobby, the taxation on horses lobby, the company lobby … and really maybe what we are saying is that the married professional couples' lobby is not as powerful yet to force a change.'

Frequently in the debate, Kate comes across as being detached, even though she herself is a victim of the tax system under discussion. Not for the first time, Murphy seems to mistake her impartiality for indifference. From it he infers that she believes that 'it is not entirely desirable to make a change to the system' – but he is mistaken.

'I did not say it is not entirely desirable to make a change,' she shoots back. 'I think it is very possible with the political will to do so,' and she immediately hits her mark in her suggestion that the Australian system, which taxes people as separate individuals, should be considered as an option.

As Kate watches the debate, she smiles when the often volatile exchanges between the panellists are punctuated by bursts of humour. I notice that she is amused when, on the screen, she chides Divaris for being 'naughty' for his cheeky suggestion that some married women, who are unhappy with the tax system and unhappily married, could change their circumstances *and* thereby pay less tax and lose their husbands at the same time. Does she appreciate, I wonder, the incisive practical insight of the woman who refuses to let Divaris get away with his glib suggestion?

When he suggests that women could submit separate tax assessments, she counters, 'You can have separate assessments, but Costa knows very well that the amount of tax paid is exactly the same. Most women are not very fussed about whether they are disappearing as individuals; they just do not like the lumping of income together, and that it costs them money. The family bill is the same, and that is the issue.'

As we continue to watch, Kate – who has become for me Kate-on-the-screen as opposed to Kate-on-the-sofa – seems to dominate the debate. When Murphy asks her if she accepts that the government is tackling the issue in as 'fast and as rational' a manner as it can, she gives him a dismissive, withering look, and says, 'That is a very difficult question to ask someone who is on the Standing Commission. All I can say is that having got involved in looking at tax issues for the past four years, I realise how many lobbies there are, and how difficult it is to pick your way through them. The government has lots of lobbies to answer to all the time.'

Kate's onscreen performance reaches new heights when the discussion turns to some of the secondary consequences of South Africa's tax regime, and Sue Grant and Carmen Nathan veer off at a tangent about the 'immorality' of couples living together instead of marrying in order to avoid excessive tax.

Kate will have none of it. 'Nigel,' she interjects, with all the moral authority of a woman whose argument is incontrovertible in the South African context of the day, 'on the moral issue, it is a very dangerous argument because I think while we all do know someone who is living with someone else for tax reasons – though I am not sure how widespread it is – I think tax has less to do with morality than the price of bread has to do with morality, and if you start asking the government to start making changes in tax for moral reasons, it is dangerous because we invite them to intervene in other areas too, and there is far too much meddling by the authorities in the morals and values of this country.'

Kate's rebuttal of her fellow panellists' emotive arguments moves Murphy to jest, 'I am not sure which side of the fence you're on!'

Kate smiles, but is unfazed by the suggestion that she's breaking ranks, and she goes on to respond: 'I am in favour of change for rational economic reasons. I find it dangerous when you start bringing moral issues in.'

I cannot help but wonder, at this point, whether it is the discipline of her mathematical training that enables her to separate issues with such lucidity, to express herself so unambiguously.

Murphy returns to the central issue of the possibility of changing the system, but Kate retorts with a hint of impatience: 'Of course it's possible.' And when Murphy quips in response, 'That some acceptable compromise will be found?', Kate sits back in her chair and says, 'That's for the politicians to decide ... always.' She returns to what is clearly, for her, a basic consideration: whatever change is made, it should not penalise working couples in the lower-income groups. With an incredulous look on his face, Murphy replies, 'If you can see this way through the morass, why are you not suggesting it?' Clearly peeved and puzzled, Kate smartly responds, 'Why are you assuming that I am not?'

The debate is all but over, and Murphy has no time to engage Kate on this point. In summing up, though, she has the last word: 'I think we must accept the principle that a husband and wife are separate individuals and deserve separate treatment as taxpayers. Once you've accepted that, you can look at the options.'

The *Midweek* theme tune signals the end of the programme and fuzzy snow appears on the screen. The image of Kate-on-the-screen, in full cry, remains with me: her grasp of issues, her fine debating ability, and, despite her occasional annoyance at some of the more obtuse points made, her generosity in dismissing the unsound arguments of certain fellow panellists in the nicest way.

Her ability to be forcefully opinionated intrigues me, for she would often raise her voice just enough to complete her argument, though without compromising her position on the Standing Commission, at all times offering a clear, unemotional view of the political and economic dynamics of taxation.

In a newspaper report at the time on the lively exchange of ideas on the programme, Kate Jowell is singled out as being 'a particularly formidable debater': 'It may sound odd to draw an analogy between her and a boxer, but that is how she came across – standing aloof from the initial flurry of exchanges, then stepping in and picking her verbal punches with telling effect.'[252]

Kate-on-the-sofa, who has long stopped watching the screen but seems to be thinking about her television performance, says, with apparent self-irony, 'I'd buy a used car from that woman!' Together, we burst out laughing. I had hoped to talk to Kate about her current views, two decades later, on the role of women in society today, on how life is different – or the same – for her two daughters. For they, too, will have 'two jobs' if they choose to pursue a career once they get married: one at home, and one at work.

But it is all too clear that Kate is not able to discuss the debate or expand on her theories, her hopes, her disappointments. I realise that I somehow expected a miracle, and I mask my dismay, my growing sense of sadness for the predicament of this woman. We talk briefly about the artworks on the walls of my lounge, and then I disappear into the kitchen to put the kettle on.

Ivan will soon be here to take her home.

12

Superwoman

(1983–85)

T HE BOOK'S SPINE, once a tart tangerine, has faded over the years to a dull mustard colour. Flecks of white scar the cover, and tell-tale creases indicate that the well-thumbed Penguin paperback has been read, and reread. I am scanning Kate Jowell's bookcase in the Glencoe Road study – a fascinating exercise – for clues to her character, to the things that interested, inspired and intrigued her – when *Superwoman* catches my eye.

The title of Shirley Conran's bestselling 'bible' on household management that revolutionised the homes and lives of millions of women in the 1970s and 1980s is legible – but only just. Kate's copy is the South African edition, with an introduction by her erstwhile colleague and friend, Jane Raphaely. I dip into it, trying to imagine Kate poring over it, and wondering what she made of it all, especially the section titled 'How to be a Working Wife and Mother'. For Kate herself was more than qualified to write that chapter.

By 1984, her husband was fast becoming one of South Africa's top businessmen: Trencor was thriving under Neil Jowell's direction. And her little girls were growing up – Justine was nine years old, Nicola was six. Was their childhood happy and carefree? I wonder. Who helped them with their homework? Who brushed their hair in the mornings? Who played Snakes and Ladders with them? Who taught them to tie their shoelaces? Kate would surely have done these things, and more, when she was at home in the evenings on weekdays, and at weekends. She was a loving and devoted mother, but her demanding career often took her away from home, and from her girls, and so they were left in the care of other people – their nanny, or their father, when he was home.

'Both our parents used to travel quite a bit,' Justine tells me, 'and we didn't always know where they were. You don't, when you're a child.'[253] She says this somewhat phlegmatically, without a trace of regret, but it must have stung her when she was small, and perhaps her independent spirit is a result of having had to deal, at such a young age, with the physical absence of her mother – and sometimes her father, too.

Justine's recollection of her childhood is vague. She remembers that Kate loved to play the piano, and often played for her and Nicola. 'We had a songbook, and she'd play for us and we'd sing.' Christmas and Easter celebrations stand out in her mind as special times, as do her and Nicola's birthdays. 'Ma always used to make a huge effort for our birthdays. We always had a party, and such special cakes. I remember having a "Maya the Bee" cake one year,' she says.

There are happy snaps of the children's birthday parties in the family album. I recall Kate admitting rather ruefully while I was paging through it one afternoon with her and Justine that, while she herself had ordered the impressive cakes, she had, in fact, not baked them. 'Don't worry, Ma,' Justine quickly reassured her at the time, 'we always regarded them as your cakes, no matter who did the baking.'

Kate was certainly involved in her children's lives. Her bookshelves reveal that she put a lot of thought into rearing her daughters, from the time they were born through their toddler years and later, when they were adolescents and young adults. Kate's copy of the classic handbook for parents, *Baby and Child Care* by Dr Benjamin Spock, has been referred to so many times that it is practically falling apart.

She also consulted another guru at the time, psychiatrist Dr DW Winnicott, whose classic, *The Child, the Family, and the Outside World*, was clearly one of her staples when she needed inspiration or direction on mothering her girls. Winnicott coined the classic phrase, 'the good enough mother' – and this must surely have comforted Kate as she strove for perfection in all aspects of her life, mothering included.

There are many other similar titles on the shelves, including *Your Child's Room* by Lena Larsson, and this comprehensive little library on childcare discloses, behind the high-powered Kate Jowell of the time, a dedicated mother – in spite of the fact that she often mothered her girls from a distance.

Justine tells me that she 'didn't really mind' that Kate worked long hours. But after a moment of silence she concedes, 'In retrospect, I *must* have missed her … it's difficult formulating my thoughts today.'[254] And, I silently surmise, difficult to conjure up the confusion of feelings that children so often experience when parents are absent.

Of the two girls, Justine had the easier relationship with Kate, 'especially during adolescence'.

'There was a lot of rivalry between me and my sister, and I think that Nicola felt that Ma took my side. I don't know if Ma really did take my side … maybe it just seemed that way to Nicola.' Nicola, Justine believes, 'found some things really hard'. Clearly, Kate's frequent trips away and her busy working life affected Nicola deeply. Justine continues: 'My sister struggled a bit at school, especially in early high school, and I think it was hard for her, seeing as our parents were both super-achievers.'

Certainly, to both girls, their parents must have seemed omniscient and omnipotent, for Kate and Neil Jowell were in a class of their own.

Today, their daughters are consistently loyal to both parents, and certainly to their 'ma', of whom they are obviously very proud. Justine tells the story of how a schoolmate once asked Nicola, in the disarmingly direct way of a child, 'Are you rich?' After reflecting on the question for a minute, Nicola replied, 'Yes, my mom owns all the money.'

When Kate heard about the incident, she laughed and explained to her youngest daughter that she didn't, in fact, 'own all the money', and that her salary as a business academic was somewhat less than that of her husband, the CEO of a family transport empire. Some time later, I hear another version of this story – from Neil, who gives it a slightly different angle. The rather poignant anecdote has clearly become part of the family's personal mythology.

A super-successful self-made woman, Kate Jowell probably chafed a little at earning less than her husband. But while she was positive and assertive about where she was and where she wanted to be, she was also realistic about the challenges that she and other working women faced. When *Fair Lady* asked her why women executives were so heavily out-numbered by their male counterparts, she explained that a basic problem was society's failure to assist women in handling two demanding jobs simultaneously.

'If you look around the world at women executives,' she said, 'a large number are either single or childless, and don't have to balance so many major roles.'[255] She pointed out that the responsibility of child-rearing and homemaking 'still falls unevenly on the woman ... and even if work-ing women do have help in the home, they still carry the main emotional and practical burden of seeing that things get done properly'.

Even though her own personal financial circumstances enabled her to hire domestic help, Kate was acutely aware that it was difficult for career women to 'have it all' if they did not enjoy the resources that were at her disposal. 'It's no wonder that some women actually avoid executive appointments because, at certain periods of their lives, they can't handle the dual responsibility of job and family.'

This understandable response was often regarded, by the women themselves and by society, as an admission of failure. 'And to complicate matters, many women are conditioned into thinking that if they don't perform superbly on the home front despite holding a demanding job, they're not "real" women.'

However, she also suggested that women often scuppered their chances of getting to the top of their professions because they were con-cerned, subconsciously, about whether it was appropriate for them to pursue a career in a field perceived to be the traditional domain of men. 'Their own confusion about what constitutes femininity can sometimes stop them from being positive and assertive about where they want to be – and go. They don't ask for opportunities, so they tend to get over-looked,' Kate observed, refusing to make excuses for her gender. 'The result is more frustration with their careers and, sometimes unfairly, more blame heaped on the sexual discrimination pile.'[256]

Again, we hear Kate speak her mind with confidence and cool logic. Her comments have a particular resonance today, when women's oppor-tunities to take up management positions are more advantageous than they've ever been. And it's likely that the effect of her words will be as intimidating to many women today as they no doubt were twenty years ago. Kate's vocabulary has never included the word 'victim'. Her approach was always considered and fair, and she never sided with other women simply out of a sense of loyalty.

Kate dismissed the notion of dressing for success, for when women aped men in business suits, it only confused the issue. 'Unless you are comfortable with yourself and your own style, such clothes will remain little more than a disguise.' Success, she said, had no gender, and the sooner women accepted this, and made the most of themselves 'as people rather than as imitation men', the faster they'd climb the corpo-rate ladder.[257] This was certainly her personal credo, and the way she carefully orchestrated her metamorphosis from Kathy Bowman to Kate Jowell is a telling outward reflection of her inner resolve to do just that: make the most of her own unique talents.

What is refreshing about her approach, and perhaps another reason why she alienated many women, is that she refused to lambaste men simply for the sake of doing so. She recognised and acknowledged their strengths, especially when it came to their ability to succeed.

Drawing on her own experience, she believed that women had 'some advantages in business, because they are something of a novelty and per-haps get more attention'. This also meant, however, that women were subject to careful scrutiny. 'Problems a woman may have are ascribed to her femaleness rather than her personality or ability. Prejudiced people may believe she overreacts because she's a woman, not because she's impulsive by nature.'

As in the broader labour arena, Kate appealed for changes in the way society was structured – but she never fell back on the convenience of gender stereotyping as a way out for women. 'We need empathy, tolerance and the urge to so structure our society as to give everyone the opportunity to maximise their talents and get the most out of their lives.'[258]

In many respects, Kate herself was the perfect role model. She had maximised her own talent to great effect. But she would not have been able to do this without her husband's support, and she must certainly have had Neil in mind when she commented that 'an approving man in a woman's life may play a decisive role in helping her feel comfortable with her career ambitions. Supportive fathers, husbands and boyfriends, who take pleasure in seeing a woman working and achieving in whatever field she chooses, are great confidence builders.'[259]

By 1984, Kate Jowell was one of South Africa's most visible women executives. The media perpetuated the image that top career women were tough superwomen who had mastered the art of juggling families and careers. Kate didn't subscribe to the view that women who were at the top were brittle and bitchy, with a killer instinct to match. Rather, she believed that a key quality in women is the ability to inspire and motivate other people.[260] She reasoned that there were so few top women executives because women were trying to make their way in a working environment 'made by men for men'. She reiterated her old theme: 'We should try and redesign the working environment to accommodate women's needs.'

Her perception was that many women were not conditioned to succeed and did not therefore feel comfortable in top management positions. Others, however, felt unable to cope with the overload of running a family and holding an executive position. In a rare moment of speaking from the heart, Kate Jowell admitted, 'What is exhausting is handling the responsibility at work and then going home to another set of executive decisions. At a certain point with children, women can feel torn into 10 000 pieces.'[261]

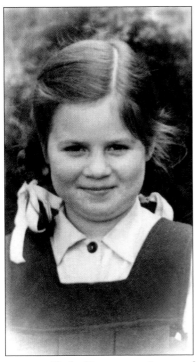

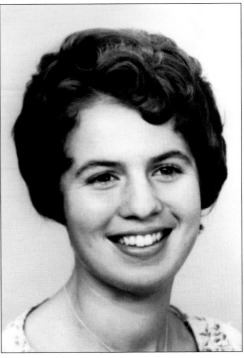

Kathy Bowman at the age of
six and a half, June 1946

Kathy, circa 1959

© Werner's Studios

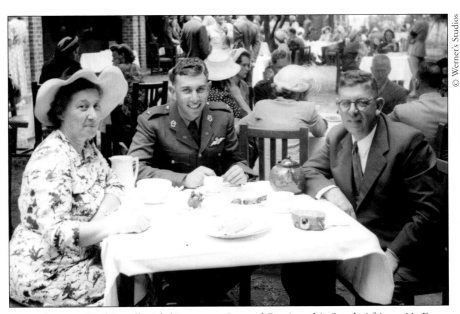

A young Neil Jowell with his parents Joe and Bessie at his South African Air Force
passing-out parade in Pretoria, February 1952

FROM KATHY JOWELL, EDITOR

INSIDE

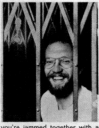

'IT'S AN anti-women-liberation thing — I've put the woman back in her cage,' Jac de Villiers says facetiously. He's the clever photographer who caught our fashion feature on page 90 between floors as the models zipped up and down in lifts — or elevators as they have it in America. 'I've always been fascinated by lifts — suddenly you're jammed together with a whole bunch of people you don't know. It's kinda tense.' Jac's been photography-mad since he was 12. He had a brief spell at the University of Cape Town studying Civil Engineering before returning to the craze full time — working initially for photographer Beresford McNally. 'Beresford is a wizard at technique and I learnt a lot in the two years we worked together.' Now Jac goes it alone with a camera and a bag of talent. 'I love photographing women, trying to capture that elusive quality of femininity...' Which he does, sensitively. Next year he intends going to live and work in London — doing photography and also a course in graphic design. And keeping women — for the present — firmly on the other side of his lens ...

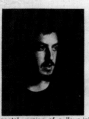

RENÉ HERMANS started as a printer in Holland, graduated to an advertising agency and has now reached nirvana as a freelance commercial artist in Cape Town, where he has lived for eight years. Nirvana also includes his marriage to Maureen England of '8 Birds/8 Beasts' fame. They met on a 'heap sleep' which we're told is a horizontal version of a 'love-in' — clearly an appropriate place to meet one's future spouse! 'Maureen and I have completely different interests and by the time I've got

books and children. It's an ambition in keeping with his relaxed attitude to life: 'I'll never get steamed up trying to be rich and rare, just so long as I'm happy.'

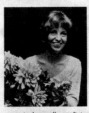

MADELEINE DOBSON our newest editorial secretary has taken our appearance firmly in hand. Here she puts the finishing touches to the office flower bowl which has never had it so professional. When she was in Hong Kong she took a course in Ikebana (Japanese flower arranging). 'I only did it for a couple of months and it takes seven years to be really proficient,' she says modestly. Madeleine got her taste for travel early when she left Canada with her parents to settle in England. Her working life has been split between many countries — England, Canada,

remained
FAIR LA
that inte
much dit
can tip t
she's b
such as
for her
things a
intereste
drama. V
office to keep anyone entertained. Who needs footlights as well?

KATHY BOWMAN
Assistant Editor

fair lady
THE MAGAZINE FOR MODERN WOMEN

P.S. BOX 1802 · CAPE TOWN · PHONE 41-3141 · TELEGRAMS "LADYFAIR"

IT'S TIME to e
and end on a n
I will have left
years. It's been
birth of a new
monthly to for
size, and final
square-back bi
editor have b
contact with ne
— by phone, in print, often face-to-face and especially through your letters — has made this if not a hot seat,
and satisfying one! I'm sad to
ve a soft spot for the magazine
just a job, and for the colleagues
om FAIR LADY's success would
e and thank you for being such
great knowing you ...

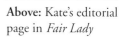

Kathy Jowell
Editor

Fair Lady

LEEUSIG, 4 LEEUWEN STREET
P.O. BOX 1802 · CAPE TOWN · TEL. 3-6886

Above: Kate's editorial page in *Fair Lady*

Left:
Kate (second from right) at a *Fair Lady* function. Beauty editor Peggy Page is on her right, and photographer Volker Milos is seated next to Peggy

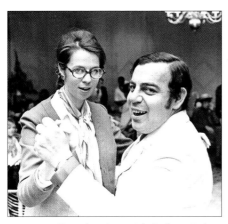

Kate dancing with Sydney Baker,
Fair Lady's legendary fashion editor

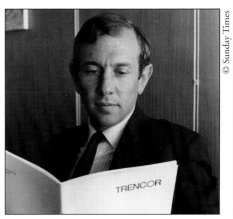

© Sunday Times

Neil Jowell at the Trencor head office
in Cape Town

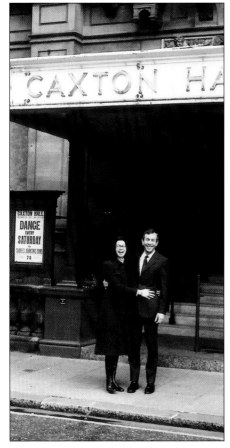

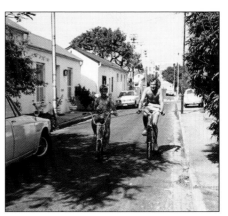

Neil and his son Michael outside Kate's
Ayres Road, Rosebank cottage, 1972

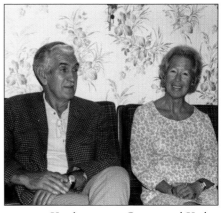

Neil and Kate on their wedding day,
8 October 1970, at the Caxton Hall
registry office in London

Kate's parents, George and Kathy,
at Sheerness in Kent, July 1972

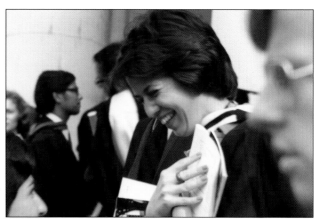

Right:
A new beginning:
Kate graduated with an
MBA from the UCT
Graduate School of
Business in June 1974

© The Argus

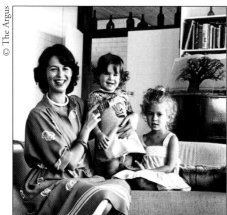

Kate, Nicola and Justine at home in
Gardens, circa 1979

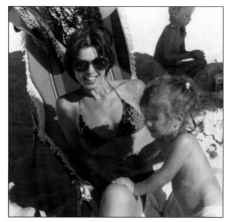

Kate and Nicola on Clifton Beach, 1980

© Rosemarie Frey

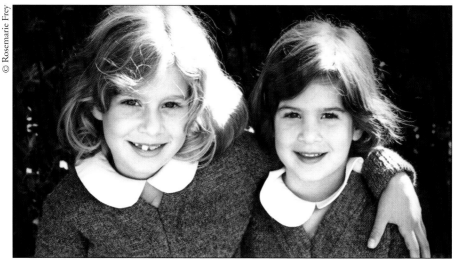

The Jowell girls

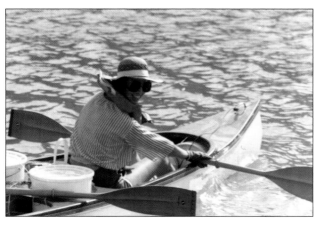

Left:
Kate on the Orange River, scene of many happy family holidays

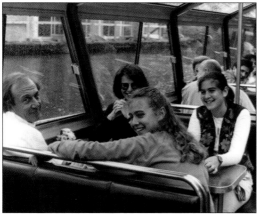

The Jowell family on holiday in Amsterdam, 1990

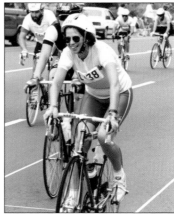

Kate participating in the 1991 Cape Argus Pick 'n Pay Cycle Tour

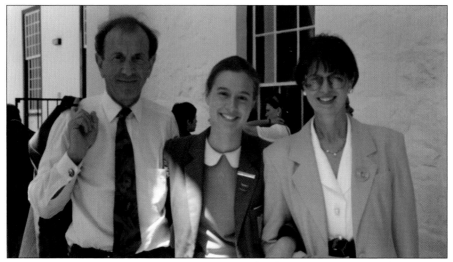

Neil and Kate at Justine's valediction, 1993

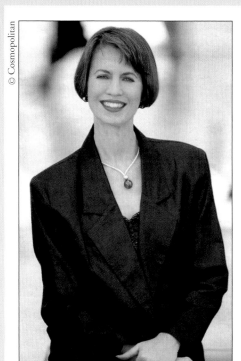

© Cosmopolitan

Left:
Kate at the pinnacle of
her career, 1993

Below:
A stylish Kate delivering
a speech at a Cape Town function

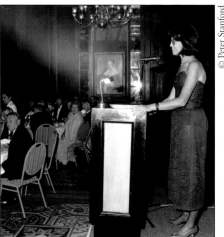

© Peter Stanford

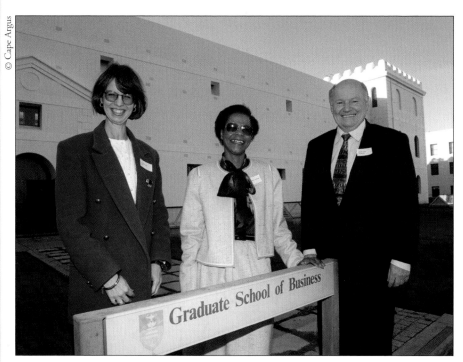

© Cape Argus

The GSB Breakwater Campus at the Victoria & Alfred Waterfront.
With Kate are Mamphela Ramphele and Mike Levett, 1996

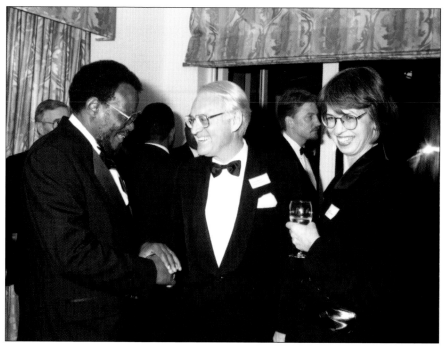

Kate with Mangosuthu Buthelezi and Denis Worrall at a GSB dinner on 29 August 1996

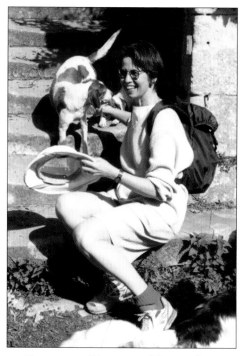

Kate on a walking tour of the Dordogne in 2000, when her health took a turn for the worse

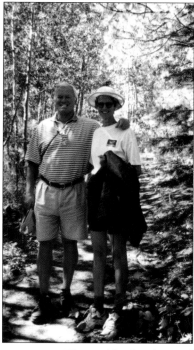

Kate and her brother Paul at Lake Nevada, 2002

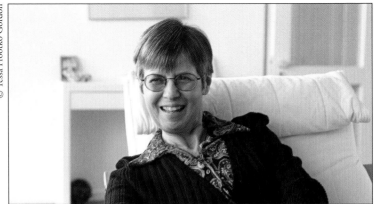

© Tessa Frootko Gordon

Kate in 2003. These are the last photographs taken of her

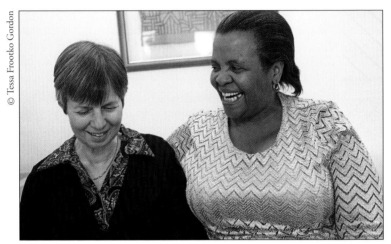

© Tessa Frootko Gordon

Kate with her caregiver Eunice Mzondi at the time
her life story was being recorded, 2003

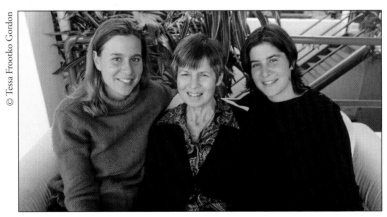

© Tessa Frootko Gordon

Kate and her daughters Justine and Nicola, 2003

Kate's comment is more than a little revealing: there must have been occasions – when her children were ill, or when they had a problem or a prize-giving – that her loyalties were divided. Inevitably, she must have been forced to compromise at times, playing off certain demands against others that may have appeared less important at a given moment.

Yet for all this, life at Glencoe Road was as interesting as it was adventurous. In the mid-1980s, the cul-de-sac had very few houses and, given its dramatic position, with Table Mountain looming over it, the wildness of the setting would have inspired imaginative children's games and an exciting sense of freedom. At that time, the Jowells decided to buy the adjoining plot, and started building their dream home – the one they live in today.

The house's design is simple, the kind of simplicity that, from the street level, appears ordinary, and even banal. But it is a deceptive first impression, for, as all good buildings should, the house capitalises superbly on the attributes of the site, its steepness, its heart-stopping views of the sea, and the imposing backdrop of the mountain.

But in 2003, like its mistress, the house is a shadow of its former self. Kate restlessly wanders around inside it. The grand dinner parties of former years have shrunk to occasional family suppers. This is no longer a place where people are entertained, stimulated, nurtured. Even though the house is light and airy, an air of illness clings to its walls, rendering it sombre and soulless. And it is only at night, when the twinkling lure of the city below casts a seductive glow and the television chatters away with Neil and Kate watching, that the house regains something of its past aura.

~

In 1983, Kate Jowell continued to speak out against South Africa's unjust political system and its disastrous effect on workplace dynamics. When asked in an interview whether the substantial increase in strikes since 1979 was 'an alarming development', she observed that this was not necessarily a bad sign.[262]

South Africa was still relatively strike-free. But, she cautioned, 'rather than congratulating ourselves on not having strikes, we should look at the social cost we paid to avoid them'. Though some believed that the labour relations system had served the country well in the past because of the relative paucity of strikes, Kate said that the situation should be looked at from the perspective of the people whom it did *not* serve. She pointed out that 'labour docility [had been bought] at a high social cost – in poor working conditions, lack of opportunity, poor productivity, the social consequences of security police action, and so on'.

She believed that strikes should be decriminalised, and that one of the most positive aspects of the revival of black trade unionism was that, for the first time, black unions were 'forcing white management to sit around the table with blacks and try to establish a relationship based on some kind of equality'.

Kate saw that even though certain prejudices were being confirmed in the process, others were being eroded, and a mutual understanding was developing between the two groups. She was able to express an optimism that would later be confirmed: 'I'm immensely hopeful that this kind of political change towards attitudes and practices will ultimately help to speed [up] major political reform.'[263]

But the reform she had in mind was certainly not the political change PW Botha engineered for the country in 1983. The introduction of a new Constitution provided for a tricameral – or three-chamber – parliament to accommodate qualified political representation for coloureds and Indians, while, for the second time in a century, the political rights of the black majority were ignored.

The Minister of Constitutional Affairs, Chris Heunis, plainly stated the objective of the Constitution: it granted rights to coloureds and Indians 'without detracting from the self-determination of the whites'.[264]

There was a hunger for change in the early 1980s. It was obvious to white South Africa that preserving minority rule would come at an ever-increasing cost. The questions were how much change would the white electorate accept as necessary, and would the changes appease the government's increasingly vociferous critics? Judging from the referendum in November 1983 – when two thirds of the 76 per cent of whites who turned out to vote backed the proposal – the new Constitution was seen by the white minority as a step in the right direction.

But sentiments beyond the suburbs were very different. Intensified resistance to what was seen as mere tinkering rather than fundamental reform gave rise to two new extra-parliamentary groupings: the ANC-affiliated United Democratic Front (UDF) and the National Forum (NF), which aligned itself with the Black Consciousness Movement (BCM).

While the insufficiency of Botha's reforms inflamed the left, the reforms were regarded as radical and unacceptable by conservative elements in his own party, some of whom had gone so far as to break away in 1982 to form the Conservative Party.

So, while the new constitutional order elevated Botha to a position of unrivalled power as formal and executive head of state, he was embattled, facing stiffening opposition from both the left and the right. And as the violent 1980s wore on, it became increasingly obvious that the 'major political change' of Kate Jowell's vision had yet to be embraced.

The times were tense, to say the least. In 1983, four months before the Constitution was approved by Parliament, a 60-kilogram bomb, hidden in a stolen car, detonated prematurely outside the headquarters of the South African Air Force in Church Street, Pretoria. More than twelve people died, and 180 were injured. It was, one survivor noted, 'a scene from hell'.[265]

The ANC accepted responsibility for the blast – claiming that the intended target had not been civilians, but the Air Force offices. Then, on the day that the new Constitution came into force, on 3 September 1984, nine people were killed in unrest in and around Sharpeville, the township where sixty-nine people had been killed by police twenty-four years earlier. A month later, 800 000 workers at key parastatals such as Iscor and Sasol staged one of the biggest stayaways South Africa had ever experienced.

Moreover, a new militancy was emerging among black trade unions. One of the most powerful of these was the National Union of Mine-workers (NUM), which was led by a young lawyer, Cyril Ramaphosa.

NUM was instrumental in initiating talks to unify the trade union movement, and towards the end of 1985 the Congress of South African Trade
Unions (Cosatu) – a giant federation representing half a million workers
at the time – was formed.

Kate Jowell keenly analysed these labour developments. She sought
out Ramaphosa to gauge his views on key labour issues, and was impressed
by him, Neil says.[266] 'His attention to detail, and his rapport with NUM
members and other key players, struck her at the time,' he recalls.

But her focus also included other issues of the day. Using every opportunity that presented itself, she urged women to organise themselves
on a large scale if they wanted to succeed in changing the joint taxation
system. Addressing a women's club in Cape Town, she noted that women
had not yet proved themselves to be a significant pressure group.[267] 'The
authorities will only respond to concerted organised pressure. They are
unlikely to change anything until it is proved that the price of maintaining the present system is greater than the price of change.'

She reiterated her belief that when a wife's income was deemed to
be part of her husband's, her independence, privacy and equality were
compromised. But she conceded that it was a very sensitive issue, one
which many women themselves had not resolved. 'Where deep-seated
values are concerned,' Kate argued, 'it's wise to move slowly. Women
are going to have to try to change things using patience, persuasion
and tact.'

In November 1984, Professor Kate Jowell was one of a nineteen-
member commission appointed by the government to overhaul the tax
system. The Commission of Inquiry into the Tax Structure of South
Africa was chaired by Mr Justice Cecil Margo, and Minister of Finance
Barend du Plessis gave the commission eighteen months to compile
a report and recommendations on taxation 'viewed from the widest
possible financial and economic perspective'.[268]

Margo assured South Africans that they could depend on the commission 'to give fearless advice based on a ruthless examination of the
facts. We are nobody's "yes-men".'[269] He believed that one of the most

important tasks of the commission was to determine how to make taxation equitable and neutral. Married women's tax, among other pressing issues, would certainly be on the agenda.

When the Margo Commission – as it soon became known – was announced, the *Sunday Times* observed that its commissioners included 'the best legal, academic, economic and business brains in South Africa'. Kate Jowell, who together with Margaret Lessing was one of two women on the commission, was in excellent company. Among the members was the Jowells' friend, Dr Jannie Graaff, who at the time was a member of the Economic Advisory Council.

'I was overseas doing some academic work when the commission was appointed, and when I returned I discovered that Kate and I would serve together,' Graaff recalls.[270] In order to 'catch up', Graaff lunched with the Jowells at Glencoe Road on his return. Kate briefed him on the commission's proceedings thus far, and gave him a sketch of their fellow commissioners. 'Her perceptions were spot-on,' Graaff later noted with an approving smile.

For the next eighteen months, Kate and Jannie Graaff would spend much time in Pretoria, where the commission sat for two to three days every week. Endorsing a view expressed by Neil Jowell, Graaff says that despite Kate's not being a tax expert, she was very interested in the effect of taxes on the labour market.

Kate's interest soon shifted to broader gender-related issues. She had been influenced by the single-mindedness of a particularly impressive adviser to the commission: Professor June Sinclair of the Law Faculty of the University of the Witwatersrand.

Commenting on Kate Jowell's contribution to the commission, Graaff commends her for her talented performance, especially in committee situations: 'She was articulate; she definitely understood the subject being discussed. People liked and respected her, so they listened to what she had to say.'

Kate's major contribution to the committee's final recommendations was on the subject of the separate taxation of married women. The recommendations were contained in a 456-page report, which was presented to President PW Botha on 20 November 1986. Chapter 7 of the report dealt specifically with the taxation of married women. Among the recommendations of the commission was that separate taxation of spouses be made compulsory, and that men and women be treated equally: 'The fundamental premise of a tax system for South Africa in the late twentieth century, the commission believes, ought to be the recognition of individual effort.'[271]

Kate's own efforts did not go unnoticed. On 18 December 1986, commission chairman Mr Justice Margo wrote her a letter of thanks for her valuable contribution. Commenting on the fact that the commission had at times been forced to work under difficult conditions, he said that it was nevertheless always a pleasure listening to Kate's submissions and evaluating her reasoned arguments. Significantly, he said, 'It is a tribute to your tact and tolerance that our differences were all resolved.'

He thanked Kate in particular for her chairing of the panel discussion that dealt with the taxation of married women, for the benefit of her experience and expertise, for her 'fearlessly independent approach', and for the crucial information she made available regarding black perceptions.

At about the same time as her appointment to the Tax Commission, Kate's tenure as a National Manpower Commission member was extended for another four-year term. Her participation in this forum was, however, not lauded in all circles. Inevitably, unionists felt that her high-profile government appointments aligned her with the state, and that they compromised her position at the University of Cape Town – widely perceived as a liberal institution in conflict with the government of the day and its dubious agenda. One union even went so far as to blackball the Business School, citing Kate Jowell's membership of the Manpower Commission as the reason.

Kate took the criticism in her stride. The commission, which was an advisory body on labour law reform and other labour matters, had a brief from government, but this was 'unexceptional', she claimed.[272] The commission had not been given a particular ideological mandate, and she therefore felt comfortable about the role she was fulfilling.

'Certainly, some of the labour reforms I wanted to see have come to pass,' she said. 'Of course, once you are involved in a body like that you have to grit your teeth when matters are decided that you don't agree with. But, up to now, enough of what I would like to see happening is happening.'

She did acknowledge, though, that her appointment had raised eyebrows in certain circles, but to her it was all simply 'a matter of perception'. Her association with the university had no bearing on her work for the commission, and she impatiently dismissed any notion to the contrary. 'The only comments I have had are that I do my homework and I fight for things I believe in. Whether or not people see me as slanting the commission in a way they wouldn't like, I don't know.' She had also not heard any gripes from the university – and asserted that she did not expect to.

'After all,' she pointed out, 'the role of a university and its academics is to gain expertise and knowledge to serve the community.'[273]

~

August 2003. The pale Cape Town sky is clear. Wisps of cloud cling to the cusp of Table Mountain. I am making my way to the Victoria & Alfred Waterfront hotel where Paul Bowman and his wife, Carina, are staying. Up till now, my contact with Kate's brother, who lives in Florida in the United States, has been limited to long-distance calls and email exchanges. Anxious about Kate's advancing Alzheimer's, he has come to see her.

Having often scrutinised the many photographs Kate has of her only sibling, I recognise Paul easily when I track him down in the hotel dining room, about to have breakfast with Carina, who has yet to arrive. An expansive, dapper man, Paul Bowman is, in many ways, the antithesis of his sister – ebullient and spontaneous, where she is discreet and measured. But there is a genuine niceness about him that Kate has in abundance too.

It is nine months since his last visit to Cape Town, and this physical and temporal interval has amplified for him the deterioration in Kate's condition. The smile on his face fades soon after our initial pleasantries, and, clearly concerned about his sister, Paul's mood darkens as he speaks.

'I was terribly upset when I saw her this week,' he starts. 'She can't put sentences together the way she used to, her spatial perception is also worse, and her incontinence, which she is refusing to acknowledge, is a terrible problem for her.'[274] Paul's face bears a pained expression. 'This disease is unbelievably cruel. I have never seen anything like it.' Carina, his wife of forty years, joins us. She is petite and pixie-like, a stylish and attractive woman.

The couple had dined with Neil and Kate the previous evening at Rozenhof, a favourite restaurant of the Jowells in the city centre. What should have been a pleasurable outing for Kate had, however, turned into an ordeal, right from the start. Paul noticed that she struggled to climb the few steps to the restaurant's front door, and during the course of the evening, she 'didn't really connect' with anyone.

'She doesn't seem great emotionally,' Paul sadly observes. 'She seems down in the dumps.' This is scarcely surprising, though, for Carina describes how, later in the evening, Kate had to endure the humiliation of needing her help in the ladies' room.

They tell me about Kate's two-week visit to their home in Sarasota, Florida, in 2002. At the time, Kate did not realise, or at least acknowledge, the extent of her own disorientation. But Paul recalls that she was still able to read then – she was in the process of completing Arthur Golden's *Memoirs of a Geisha* – and she could socialise with her hosts. 'She walked a lot, and she swam, but she got into difficulties in the sea one day and panicked, and Carina had to go in after her. I think she was quite shaken by the incident, and she didn't go near the water after that, nor did she take long walks,' Paul recalls.

Every alternate evening, Kate and the Bowmans socialised with friends, and Kate seemed to cope rather well. 'She could still hold a conversation, and she was fine, as long as I helped her with the utensils,' Carina says. But, Paul remembers, Kate was happy to return home at the end of her stay. 'I remember her phoning Eunice to tell her she was on her way home. It was clear that she relied on Eunice a great deal, and that she got on well with her.'

The visit to Florida had severe consequences, however, as Lindy Smit, the social worker appointed to monitor Kate, recalls. For, on her return, Kate was so disorientated that, for the first time since being diagnosed with probable Alzheimer's disease in 1999, she could not find her way around her own home. The effect of the time differences on her body clock, the break in her routines, the loss of the security of a familiar environment, all impacted heavily on her ability to negotiate her world. 'She was never the same afterwards,' Lindy says. 'And, from that time, her ability to help herself in everyday situations has steadily decreased.'

Regular routines provide the Alzheimer's sufferer with a certain amount of predictability in the chaotic world they inhabit, and this minimises their confusion and disorientation. Routines provide a helpful and re-assuring framework. When Kate visited Paul and Carina in America, her familiar framework fell away, leaving her unsupported and vulnerable, with disastrous results.

When I first started interviewing Kate at the beginning of 2003, she could still remember the trip to Sarasota, but the detail that stuck in her muddled mind was the moment when, at the airport, a concerned Paul put her in the capable hands of an air hostess, saying, 'Please look after my sister, she's got Alzheimer's disease.' Kate cringed at the memory, of being so exposed, and felt that she had been treated insensitively, like a child. It is clear from Paul's own explanation that, however he may have bungled things, he was concerned about his sister flying home on her own. 'It was nerve-wracking putting her on the plane, and leaving her to cope on her own, so I told the air hostesses not to let her out of their sight.'[275]

Like his sister 'Kath', Paul Bowman has made the most of what life has offered him. After graduating from UCT in 1959 with a degree in physics, he left South Africa for the United Kingdom, where he landed a job in industrial engineering with Minnesota Mining and Manufac-turing. He soon tired of the English weather, though, and returned to

Cape Town, to the Strand, where he worked for African Explosives in management.

But it wasn't long before Paul became disenchanted with the job: 'I sat around all day doing nothing, and I hated it.' It is interesting to trace the trajectory of Paul's energetic career path, which parallels in many ways that of his successful sister. Driven by the desire to achieve, and inheritors of their parents' pioneering genes, both were prepared to make radical career changes, to accept the challenges that came their way.

Unsurprisingly, when the opportunity arose to join Minnesota Mining in Johannesburg, Paul took it.

It was there that he met Carina in 1963. Their story reads like a modern-day fairy tale. In spite of having different religious beliefs – she is Jewish, he is Christian – they tied the knot two months later, and four decades down the line they are still happily married. But the first seven years of their marriage were disruptive, with Paul job- and city-hopping, and having to cope with the demands of their two small children, Heidi and Daniel. 'I was an ambitious young guy,' Paul laughs, attempting to explain the couple's migration from Johannesburg to Cape Town, and then to Durban, Port Elizabeth and East London – all in the short space of seven years.

In 1970 he found his niche, when he was employed by Johnson & Johnson. 'I never looked back,' he says. 'I was operations director, then marketing director, then general manager of the consumer business in East London.' In 1977 Paul was promoted and the Bowman family moved to Asia, to the Philippines, where they lived for three years. Another move took place in 1981, when Paul was offered the position of international vice-president for Africa, the Middle East and part of Europe.

The family relocated to the Johnson & Johnson headquarters in New Jersey in the United States, the country they have called home ever since. Paul's work often brought him to Africa, and many times he visited Zimbabwe, the country of his childhood – witnessing with sadness its gradual decline at the hands of Robert Mugabe. Paul retired in 1997 and has since been doing what he refers to as his 'own thing'.

Yet a pressing concern of his remains his ailing sister, the last living member of his family. 'The only thing I can do for Kath now,' he says with some sadness, 'is to come to Cape Town as often as I can, to give her some kind of happiness.' Then suddenly he brightens and calls Kath on his cellphone.

'Is that my favourite sister?' he all but bellows into the mouthpiece. 'Guess who I'm with?' he enquires playfully. Kate fails to give the right answer, so he replies, 'I'm with Sharon, and she's picking my brain.' Quick off the mark, Kate shoots back, 'Do you have any brains?' Paul laughs, and after a short conversation, hangs up. Observing his satisfied grin, I know exactly what he's thinking: that although the inevitable will come, all is not yet completely lost.

His sister – his 'Kath' – is still with us, even if time is running out.

part five

PRIME
TIME

13

A Powerful Presence

(1985–90)

SEPTEMBER 2003. The maze, made up of dense, spindly brown branches, seems bizarrely out of place in the middle of the vast exhibition hall. It is, nonetheless, intriguing, and visitors to the Cape Town Flower Show are drawn to its entrance like clumps of iron shavings to a magnet. Once inside, it becomes clear that this is a metaphorical maze, depicting the mental confusion of people who suffer from a daunting disease – dementia. The maze is a fund-raising and awareness drive on the part of Alzheimer's South Africa, an organisation that helps sufferers, their families and caregivers to face the challenge of living with dementia.

Just before emerging from the confines of the maze, I buy a small, sturdy white candle in lieu of a donation. Cheerful beads are strung on a delicate wire that winds from the candle's base to its tip. I am given a bookmark with two inscriptions: 'Light a candle for those in the dark' and 'When you use this bookmark to find your place, remember those who keep losing theirs'.

Kate has also visited the flower show, and I feel sure she must have seen the maze. I wonder what she would have made of it all, and if the experience was a poignant passage for her. But when next we chat at Carlucci's, over my tea and her cappuccino, she remembers nothing. She can't even recall which friend had treated her to the rare outing. Suddenly, she is visibly distraught and troubled at this state of affairs, at her inability to remember the minutiae of her week.

This is nothing new, her forgetting the who, what and when of her existence. But in the past she would joke about it all, or simply shrug, seeming to throw in the towel in a good-natured way. Now, her memory lapses deeply distress her, and for the rest of our rendezvous she averts her eyes and can't seem to make eye contact, looking down or away. My eyes seek out hers, and I find myself almost stooping to try to make some connection, to will her to meet my gaze. Perhaps it is just one of those days when things unravel a bit more than usual. Usually adept at drinking her cappuccino, today she spoons the entire contents into her mouth without lifting the cup once.

We have been chatting about Neil – whom she describes as 'sensitive and shy' – and Nicola – who she says is 'out and about with the young people'.[276] The younger of the Jowell daughters has, in fact, already returned to the United Kingdom after a short visit to Cape Town to see her mother. Kate is unsure of Nicola's whereabouts. We talk about Kate's own time in London, about the lure of the city and which of its charms, cultural or other, had held her in thrall.

'I think I liked living in London,' she says tentatively, 'but I just can't recall any of it.' The Beatles, fashion label of the moment Biba, James Bond movies … nothing is crisp or clear in Kate's mind. Finally, in exasperation, she declares, 'It's so difficult to keep these things in my head.'

When I see her a few days later, I am shocked to find her bruised and rather battered. When I enquire what has happened, she appears confused. Eunice reveals that Kate had fallen down the steep staircase that leads from the entrance foyer to the lower level of the house, where there are three bedrooms – hers and Neil's, and two more for the girls – and a family room that leads onto the pool terrace. Kate's nose is blue and swollen, and there are cuts on her face, above her lip and her left eye.

When all is revealed, she acknowledges what has happened, but cannot elaborate on or explain the terror she must surely have felt as her body crashed down the stairs. She appears stoic, but I can see that she is in pain.

An elegant military chest now guards the entrance to the stairs, effectively blocking Kate's access to almost half her home and the bedroom she has slept in for two decades. She will, I assume, never go down those stairs again. She and Neil have moved their bedroom, and they're now ensconced in the upstairs en-suite guest bedroom, which is next to the study. The shrinking of her personal space is a striking turning point: her isolation is more marked now than ever before, her movements curtailed in her own home.

But she is still game for cappuccino at Carlucci's. Though I am hesitant and unsure about the exercise, she wills me to take her for our usual outing. I succumb. But the moment we leave the house, I regret not having been firm with her, or sidetracking her. Today, she battles to work out how to get into my car. And the words one normally uses to describe so mundane an action are suddenly devoid of meaning. I ask her to lift her right leg, but the word 'lift' is not making any sense to her. I try again, asking her to move her foot upwards and place it on the floor of the car. She shifts about uneasily, from one foot to the other. But her feet remain on the driveway outside my car. Finally, I try to lift one of her feet without unbalancing her, and gently ease her into the car.

When we arrive at Carlucci's, she briefly battles to hoist herself onto one of the high stools. And when her cappuccino arrives, she gives it her full attention. I am tense and nervous, fretting about the home run, about getting her back into the car. When it's time to leave, we make our way, slowly, to the car, which is parked right outside the entrance, next to the outside seating area. Kate again has the problem of trying to figure out how to get into the car. At one point, she seems suddenly to decide to sit down, right there, on the pavement. I stop her, she rights herself, and we try again. People stare at us, some with curiosity, others with sympathy and concern. But no one offers to help. In the end, I do the same thing I had done in Glencoe Road. I lift her foot and manoeuvre her into the car.

It is distressing. On arriving at the house, I question Eunice closely as to whether this kind of thing has happened before, whether Ivan Jacobus, Kate's driver, has been having the same problems. Eunice is unsure, but observes, 'The illness is getting much worse.'

It is clear that Kate is well past what David Shenk calls the middle stage of Alzheimer's, the stage that 'brings the end of ambiguity'. As Shenk explains: 'The subtle cues that something was not quite right – so easy to miss a few years ago – are now bright, self-reflecting signposts of decline, impossible to avoid. Conversation is pockmarked with lost names and empty recollections. Time and dates have become fungible. Concentration wanes. The mind is now clearly ebbing ...'[277]

Inside the brain, a precise trail of pathology marks the progression of the disease. By the second stage, the plaques and tangles have spread well beyond their starting point in the brain's hippocampus, and have 'leeched' into the temporal, parietal and frontal lobes of the cerebral cortex. Shenk offers a chilling description of this decline: 'Throughout much of the thinking brain, gooey plaques now crowd neurons from outside the cell membranes, and knotty tangles mangle microtubule transports from inside the cells. All told, tens of millions of synapses dissolve away.'[278]

The exact location of neuronal loss determines what specific abilities will become impaired – and when. The process is like a series of circuit breakers shutting down one by one. In the beginning, memory formation fails as the hippocampus starts to degenerate. Then the sufferer loses control over primitive emotions such as anger, fear and craving.

It is difficult to comprehend fully the devastating consequences of Alzheimer's, often because the cognitive abilities that decline in the middle stage of the disease are the very basic ones, the ones we take for granted. The ability to understand simple questions, gestures, instructions; the ability to follow a conversation, or even keep track of one's own words or thoughts; the ability to keep track of the days of the week, the months of the year, the hours and minutes of the clock; the ability to choose one's clothes, dress oneself, have a bath; the ability to recognise former colleagues, friends, family – even one's spouse; the capacity for awareness, awareness of a terrible condition like Alzheimer's.

'Perhaps the only practical way to understand such a catastrophic loss is to imagine oneself as a very young child who has not yet developed these abilities in the first place,' Shenk suggests.[279]

This reverse childhood analogy, of an adult traversing his or her way back to infancy, is one that rankles, and – understandably – it offends the caregivers and family members of many sufferers. It comes across as the ultimate insult. To seem to strip a parent of his or her authority is demoralising and tragic. It is children, not adults, who are regarded as 'incomplete' persons, Shenk says. 'We love them ... and recognise them as human beings but we do not fully trust them. We assume a certain responsibility and even moral superiority over them. To assume this same posture toward a parent or grandparent who has stood for a lifetime in a position of moral authority is a sad and sour thing.'[280]

It is a sad and sour thing for an outsider to observe, too. For to watch a woman one has admired have every skill, feeling and fact steadily obliterated from her mind is not only sad and sour, but also scary. Mostly, though, it is the sadness that is overwhelming.

In August 2003 the Jowell family congregated in the South of France to celebrate Neil's seventieth birthday. His sons flew in from around the world, as did Justine and her boyfriend, Ross Frylinck, and Nicola. Kate was not among them. After an initial plan to fly her to France, accompanied by Eunice (Neil was already overseas on business and would join the family there), it was decided that the long-haul flight, and the trip in general, would be detrimental to her overall well-being. She would be disorientated and confused in a foreign environment, even if she were surrounded by her husband and their children. Neil, initially determined that she should be there, eventually abandoned the idea, having been urged to do so by Kate's social worker, Lindy Smit.

And Kate, who was terribly excited at the prospect, gradually forgot all about it, and never mentioned it again. The trip came and went, and she was none the wiser.

On his return, Neil said the event 'went very well indeed'. 'Everyone enjoyed themselves. And in retrospect, it would have been impossible for Kate.'[281] I ask him what it was like for him to celebrate this milestone without her, and he replies, 'Well, by now, she has missed so many other things. But in the evenings, when everyone had gone to bed, I felt terribly sad. My sons were very nice about the fact that she was not there, though obviously they didn't feel it as deeply as the girls and I did. But everyone understood that it was for the best.'

Soon after speaking to Neil, I find a Mother's Day card from Nicola, sent decades earlier. On the cover is a picture of a lost little girl cowering next to the leg of a policeman. The inscription reads, 'Mom, I'll never forget that time we went shopping and I got lost and asked a policeman if he thought we'd ever find you and he said …'

The text continued on the inside: '… "I don't know, there are so many places to hide."' To which Nicola had added, 'Dear Mom, I don't think I want to lose you … You are the Greatest! Bye, Nicola.'

The irony of the card, that one day her clever and accomplished mother would indeed get lost, cuts deep. The year was 1988. Nicola's mother was then in her prime.

~

In the 1980s, Kate Jowell was determined to 'contribute to change and society in general'.[282] She continued to busy herself with tax and labour reforms through her membership of the National Manpower Commission and the Margo Commission. She'd been appointed a director of the Western Cape Board of Barclays Bank, and a member of the Labour Affairs Committee of the Cape Chamber of Commerce. Her specific focus remained industrial relations. She taught, and she consulted.

'I try to look at industrial relations from a nuts-and-bolts point of view,' she said at the time. 'How can you manage labour/management relations better in the workplace?' And, from a broader point of view, she was keen to explore what management as a body, a pressure group, needed to know and do to influence and change government policy.

These were difficult and dangerous times for South Africa as a whole, and also for the Nationalist government. In July 1985, President Botha, prompted by mounting township unrest, imposed a state of emergency on thirty-six magisterial districts. A month later, on 15 August, he delivered his disastrous 'Rubicon' speech, in which he arrogantly asserted that he would not 'give in to hostile pressure and agitation from abroad'. The world had been expecting Botha to 'cross the Rubicon' and announce an era of radical reform. But more than 300 million television viewers across the world watched aghast as he thundered on, with sinister veiled threats of what would happen if he and the government felt they were being pushed too far.

On the labour front, unity talks among trade union blocs resulted, in 1985, in the formation of Cosatu. Together with its affiliates, Cosatu aligned itself with the UDF and later with the ANC and the South African Communist Party (SACP). Its genesis was followed by a massive wave of strikes, the highest number of strikes in ten years.

Cosatu's formation and modus operandi had unsettled the business community, and the observations and interpretations of a labour commentator such as Kate Jowell were valued and sought after at the time.

In Kate's view, Cosatu's radical element was – as she explained to the Johannesburg alumni association branch of the Business School – ahead of its rank-and-file membership, and the radicals were not paying sufficient attention to 'seeking mandates from members for executive action'.[283] The more pragmatic leadership within Cosatu realised, she argued, that this confrontation politics posed a danger to the entire union movement unless those responsible knew how and when to beat a strategic retreat.

Kate went on to point out that unions, generally, were either reformist or radical in intent. The former worked within the economic system to reform it, using legal channels and industrial action to achieve their purpose. Radical unions, on the other hand, were keen to pursue the destruction of capitalism.

Trade union membership had increased by over 300 per cent since 1973 because of black and coloured enrolments. Kate said it was encouraging to see this shift in union composition, though she regretted that the union movement was still fragmented along racial and ideological lines.

With her eye on the future, she advised South African managers not to stay out of politics, but rather to cooperate with the appropriate unions and search for creative solutions to what she saw as a unique set of problems.[284] She examined the ideological struggle within Cosatu's populist and 'workerist' factions regarding the role of a trade union movement in the current circumstances and concluded that, since its formation, the workerist approach had by no means been crushed.

In Kate's opinion, the 'stayaway weapon' was the most important aspect of the Cosatu debate, as it brought out the differences between the two factions. The populists believed that the stayaway should be used with increasing effect 'to bludgeon Pretoria', while the workerists saw it as a weapon whose value was more symbolic than real, and the use of which should therefore be controlled and limited.

Business had, she believed, taken 'positive steps' by joining forces with some unions over forced removals, and ending the state of emergency. 'What is needed now,' she concluded, 'is a faster search for joint union/ management action beyond the factory gates.'

A year later, in 1987, Kate warned that unless management was prepared to take on political issues, the social-democratic political system that existed in South Africa would not survive into the next century. Speaking at the nineteenth annual conference of the Insurance Institute of South Africa, she said that the balance of power in the workplace had been altered in recent years due to political, legal and environmental changes in South African society. Management could no longer call the shots.[285]

For the first time in her life, Kate noted, white power – as manifested in white management – was prepared to accommodate worker power. Management was now able to negotiate on matters that ten years previously may have seemed non-negotiable. In the process, management was 'demonstrating to a huge and important group in this country that there is something to be gained by compromise'.

Kate encouraged unions and management to get together and debate whether or not they had a joint interest in extending the arena of collective bargaining so as to bring about wider political reform. For Kate, management had no option but to get into the debate – even into the negotiation.

She warned: 'If we do not as a professional or managerial group open up the possibilities of dialogue, the forming of a social partnership with labour to shake the government from below, then I'm afraid we may have to answer to our children for it.' Once again, she reiterated that management had a responsibility to galvanise itself and others, not only to keep open the debate regarding the nature of South African society, but also to get the negotiation process going – before compromise became unattainable.

The situation in South Africa was especially volatile. The late 1980s was an era of high drama for labour: when Cosatu and the UDF called a two-day stayaway in protest against the whites-only election of May 1987, Cosatu's Johannesburg offices were bombed. PW Botha was quick to threaten extra-parliamentary groups with cutting off their foreign funding.

When asked to comment on the state of affairs, and on whether the government was about to lash out at the union movement, Kate said it was very difficult to discern the government's attitude towards labour. 'You must distinguish between the government's pre-election posturing and what civil servants like Piet van der Merwe have been saying. He has been making consistently calming and steadying statements.'[286] She was sceptical about the government's threat to halt the overseas funding of unions. 'A lot of ominous things are said in this country,' she told *Finance Week*, 'but are not carried out. Nevertheless, one is obviously concerned.'

She went on to acknowledge that if her reading of the situation was incorrect, a government backlash against Cosatu would be disastrous, as, by and large, trade union activity had been carried out according to the rules set down by law. 'It would be highly counterproductive to discourage this process,' she warned.[287]

A large amount of foreign funding for unions had been spent on supporting legal action in court. Kate believed that it would be a major mistake if such funding were interfered with, as unions would then be discouraged from using the established channels for resolving disputes.

Foreign aid had also been used to train shop stewards in negotiation techniques – a process of which Kate wholeheartedly approved.

Historian Nigel Worden indicates that by 1987 South Africa had reached a stalemate. 'Politics was bogged down in violence, society was riven with mistrust, the economy was slowing, sanctions were biting hard. White society was feeling more embattled, black society angrier.'[288]

After the 1987 election, the government found itself to the left of the official opposition for the first time since 1948: the formation of Andries Treurnicht's Conservative Party led to certain abandoned positions being reoccupied. The party took with it a fair number of government supporters, in the process weakening PW Botha's Nationalist Party power base.

Commenting on the future of business after the election, Kate expressed doubts regarding the short-term impact of the election on the economy. South Africa's economic revival did not depend as much on electoral shifts as it did on what she called 'economic fundamentals'. 'If gold remains in what looks like a long-term bull market,' she said, 'if we can maintain our current account in enough of a surplus to cover our international debt without stifling growth, if we can get control of inflation and ease the burden of fiscal drag on individuals so that they can help to spend us out of a recession – these are some of the things we need to sustain a revival.' [289]

She noted, too, that it was also crucial for South Africa to inspire external and internal confidence in its stability and political changes in order to encourage the lifting of sanctions and the return of foreign investment. This, she maintained, depended on the National Party's willingness to interpret its mandate so as to accelerate reform. But it also depended on the extent of the reform, since it was essential that the majority be brought on board so that everyone could pull together. She foresaw that the 'ending of the Group Areas Act and of separate education would bring major boosts to the economy in the form of housing development and rational use of our human and physical resources'.

Clearly, the 1980s had been a decade of remarkable personal achievement for Kate. In the business and labour community, she was seen as a powerful presence.

Her activities in this sector fed into her academic career as a lecturer in Industrial Relations at the Business School, and vice versa.

According to Professor Mike Page, a former colleague who moved on to become vice-president for academic affairs and dean of business at the McCallum Graduate School at Bentley University in Waltham, Massachusetts, Kate's talents were especially evident in the late 1980s and her impact was profound. 'She was a very strong person, very definite in her opinions,' he recalls. 'She didn't come across as being stubborn, but rather as very impressive, confident, always having enormous integrity, and a very strong ethical code.'[290]

In 1987, *The Argus* newspaper ran a poll among its readers to determine a line-up of South Africa's most influential women. Kate Jowell was among the contenders, as were two other women whose paths Kate had already – and would again – cross in a challenging way: Jane Raphaely, then editor of *Cosmopolitan*, and Mamphela Ramphele, a medical doctor who was at the time associated with UCT's Department of Social Anthropology.

~

The last five years of the 1980s were marked by personal highs – but also lows – for Kate and Neil Jowell. Their careers had soared, but in their personal lives both suffered the devastating loss brought on by the death of a parent. Neil lost his mother in 1989, while Kate's father, George Bowman, had died in England in 1985.

'Kath was very upset when our father died, as they had a close relationship,' Paul Bowman remembers. 'He was cremated in England, and his ashes were brought to South Africa, and my mother kept them in her apartment when she moved to Cape Town.'[291] The Bowmans had already been living in Devon for a few years before George succumbed to cancer.

The death notice, which Kate herself had probably placed in a Cape Town newspaper, fell out of her wildly disorganised papers while I was sifting and sorting through her things one day. It was neatly cut out and pasted onto a smallish white piece of paper with the date written beneath it: 'Bowman. – George, much loved husband of Kathleen, father and granddad of Paul, Carina, Heidi and Daniel (New Jersey) and Kate, Neil, Justine and Nicola (Cape Town), died with great courage on Sunday, May 19, in England.'

Paul says his father was stoical and circumspect about his illness. 'I suspect he knew something was up, but he didn't want to burden anyone. He was not well-off any more, although they were still comfortable. He died on the British medical system.'

Recalling a telephone conversation he had with his father while on a trip to Turkey, Paul says, 'I called him in England, and he complained of terrible pains in his stomach, but he didn't say what it was. He went into hospital soon after that, and he never came out.'

Paul is visiting Cape Town, staying at his favourite home-from-home when in the city, the Cape Grace hotel. His gestures are expansive, his voice a notch louder than the low murmurs of other guests in the hotel's airy breakfast room. 'My dad was a heavy smoker,' he says, explaining his father's cancer. 'My mother smoked too, but infrequently.'

Suddenly he changes tack, revealing that the Bowman marriage had been 'turbulent', that Kathleen and George had separated in the early 1960s for about three months before getting back together. And when Paul was working in the Philippines for Johnson & Johnson in 1978, Kathleen pined for her son, and she flew out to join him and his family for a long period. 'Dad came for a while, but Mum stayed on.' He offers no other explanation, other than his mother's devotion to him, and offers no comment on what Kate may have made of her mother's desertion of her father in favour of her brother.

Kate's own insights into her parents' character and behaviour are interesting: 'My father was a mediator of sorts.'[292] Her mother she often described – matter-of-factly, rather than with disapproval – as 'wilful'.

Her mother-in-law, Bessie Jowell, she described as 'such a star ... the doyenne of Namaqualand'.[293] Kate's relationship with Neil's mother was never close, perhaps because of circumstance, and certainly because of the distance between Cape Town and the little dorp where Bessie lived in the vast arid area of the Northern Cape.

'They never really got to know one another very well,' Neil confirms.[294] Yet the first time I chatted to Kate at Glencoe Road, she offered two snippets on Bessie Jowell without any prompting. 'My mother-in-law used to drive the trucks herself that took the ore from Springbok to …' Her voice trailed off as she lost her train of thought. We had been talking about Neil, Namaqualand and the family business. 'And she used to clean the synagogue. It's from the British side … there was a lot of difficulty when my husband decided to marry me.'

Her conversation was cluttered with disparate shards of information, bits that no longer fitted together but jarred and clashed and jostled for space in her mind. During this, our first, fragmented interview in her Glencoe Road home, I asked Kate to show me round the house. On entering the study, she pointed to the twin leather-and-steel recliners placed snugly side by side in one corner and said, 'Neil's mother saw these and bought them for us.' I was immediately struck by the unlikelihood of the claim. Possibly, Kate's memory was tripping her up. It struck me as highly incongruous that the unpretentious woman whom Kate had just described would have selected these sophisticated modern pieces of furniture for her son and daughter-in-law.

But, later, Neil confirmed that his mother had, in fact, bought the recliners – but she had not chosen them.[295] 'Kate and I had seen them in London on one of our trips and brought home a brochure. When my mother accompanied my father on an overseas trip – he was going to a motor dealer's conference in Sweden – I asked her to look out for them.' Bessie found the Stockholm shop and duly showed the shop assistant the brochure. 'They didn't have an agent in South Africa so they sold them to her at cost price and she arranged to have three of them – my brother, Cecil, also wanted one – shipped to Cape Town.'

In many ways, Kate, an independent thinker and a person in her own right, shared similar traits with her mother-in-law. They were both strong women, confident, intelligent and down-to-earth, in spite of the privileges that came with being married to a Jowell man. But in other ways, Kate was the antithesis of Bessie. She was a powerful career woman, always stylish and effortlessly groomed. Bessie, on the other hand, was not concerned with her appearance. She maintained that 'Joe could not have it all – he could not have a wife who, at the drop of a hat, could throw a party for sixty people or pack a bag and leave for Cape Town with very short notice and at the same time look groomed.'[296]

But, just like her new daughter-in-law, Bessie could hold her own anywhere in the world. Lively and interesting, this formidable Jewish woman expressed exquisite tact, a kind of *noblesse oblige*. She would, on occasion, deliberately dress down to make her guests, who may not have been as smartly turned out, feel comfortable. In whatever she did, Bessie followed the dictates of her huge, humane heart.

In her book on Joe Jowell, Phyllis Jowell tells the story of a London taxi driver who mistook Bessie for a charlady, much to her amusement. Phyllis speculates that it was probably Bessie's *doek* – which she wore around her head in inclement weather, as she was inclined to develop bronchitis – that prompted the cabbie to make the faux pas.

She goes on to describe the scene: 'On one particular trip to England in the 1960s Bessie was returning home from Oxford by cab to her hotel in London, the well-known Dorchester Hotel, when the cab driver said to her, "Well, luv, you're going to London to look for a job are you? There's many jobs for char ladies there." Was his face red when, at the Dorchester Hotel, she was ushered in by the doorman!' Bessie, who could be a lot of fun, repeated this story often and 'with gusto'.[297]

Bessie remained in Springbok for seven years after Joe's death in 1973. She wished to maintain the family's presence in Springbok, for she felt 'one could not have a business in Springbok without at least one member of the family living there'. Clearly, her loyalty and commitment to Joe persisted long after he had passed away.

But Bessie's health had begun to fail. By 1980, the family realised that she had become too frail to continue living on her own so far away, and they wanted her to be nearer.[298] Not surprisingly, Bessie was reluctant to leave the town that she and Joe had made their own, where Joe had been laid to rest, and that owed so much to their vision and entrepreneurship.

Indeed, Phyllis believes that, had it not been for a surgical procedure that finally precipitated Bessie's departure from Springbok, this feisty woman would never have been persuaded to leave.

The sad reality, though, was that Bessie was not only frail, but was also losing her faculties. Who could have predicted that she and her daughter-in-law would ultimately fall prey to the same disease? Bessie Jowell returned to Cape Town at the behest of her sons because she was suffering from Alzheimer's disease. It seems an especially cruel double blow for Neil, losing first his mother, and now his wife, to Alzheimer's.

Yet Neil's experience, and therefore his memory, of his mother's Alzheimer's is cushioned by the fact that in the first years she was still in Springbok. 'It's difficult to say when she was diagnosed,' he comments. 'It was not a traumatic thing, not as much as I would have expected. She was still living in Springbok after her Alzheimer's became evident, and I was not really exposed to it.'[299]

When his mother relocated to Cape Town, to a flat in Sea Point, it was the end of an era for the Jowell family. The last Jowell had left Springbok. In Cape Town she was cared for by her constant companion, Isobel Young. Now more accessible to her youngest grandchildren, Justine and Nicola, Ouma Bessie became a feature in their lives.

'We used to visit her most Sundays,' Neil recalls. But Kate's distant relationship with Bessie remained unchanged, partly due to Bessie's condition and Kate's unrelenting work schedule. 'When my mother came to Cape Town she was already old, and Kate was very busy,' Neil explains.

I recall that in one of my own earliest conversations with Kate, at a time when she was still able to show awareness that she had Alzheimer's, she mentioned that Bessie had succumbed to the same disease that had struck her down. With her clear gaze and her light voice, Kate stated, very simply, 'She also had Alzheimer's.' Explaining that it was 'devastating', Kate couldn't, however, extrapolate, and it seemed that the irony of the situation was lost on her.

It is interesting that Neil's own recollection of the final stages of his mother's illness is somewhat blurred. Neil is uncertain as to whether or not Bessie still recognised her sons and their families towards the end of her life. He can't remember – but perhaps he does not want to. The parallels with his wife's situation are all too obvious, too painful.

Bessie died on 14 July 1987. She made her final journey to Springbok and was buried in the Okiep cemetery next to her beloved Joe. Family members and friends flew in from around the country to pay their respects to Rebecca 'Bessie' Jowell, a remarkable woman who had led a remarkable life and who was probably one of the last Jews to be buried in Namaqualand. Two years later, in 1989 – sixty years after she and Joe had first come to Namaqualand – Bessie's tombstone was consecrated. A mirror image of Joe's, it lay next to the kokerboom she had planted when her husband died. A chapter in the Jowell family history had finally closed.

~

Joe Jowell's legacy, Trencor – the company he had built in 1930 from scratch – was flourishing. In 1987, company chairman Neil Jowell won the tenth *Cape Times* Businessman of the Year award, joining the ranks of previous award recipients who included top Western Cape business executives Aaron Searll, Jan Pickard, Neal Chapman, Jack Goldin and Stuart Shub.

At the award presentation, Gordon Kling, executive editor of the *Cape Times*, said that 'low-profile Trencor' had been a top performer on the Johannesburg Stock Exchange since 1977, and in 1986 was ranked ninth-best performer over a five-year period in the *Financial Mail*'s top 100 companies.[300] Trencor achieved record profits for the fourth consecutive year in 1987, and earnings rose by 40 per cent to 154.3c a share.[301] Kling cited the *Financial Mail*'s observation that Neil Jowell had 'become known for his conservative financial bias – and for consistently producing results that are better than his predictions'.

From humble beginnings in Namaqualand, when Joe Jowell, a garage owner, started a transport company 'to replace a railway which [had] closed down', Trencor had grown into a group employing 5 000 people.

While road transport was still its core business, it also manufactured trailers, and a subsidiary manufactured shipping containers, while export earnings made a substantial contribution to profits.[302]

Accepting the award, Neil made a plea to the government to increase privatisation. He prefaced this by saying that company chairmen and executives who made political statements should make it clear whether they were doing so in a personal capacity or as head of their organisations. He had been given a mandate from Trencor to do so since its road transport interests were in competition with the public sector. There was wide consensus, he said, that the public sector was too big and had to be reduced.

Echoing Kate's sentiments, he said private business in a free economy had an important part to play in bringing increased freedom and progress to South Africa. The government had often stated its commitment to privatisation, but its efforts had been so minimal that they 'almost amounted to sub-contracting'.[303] In his view, a bold move was required to get the ball rolling.

A photograph that appeared in the *Cape Times* the following day shows a triumphant Neil with Kate at his side – an image of togetherness and success. Indeed, the caption, headed 'Successful Couple', reads: '*Cape Times* Businessman of the Year award-winner Neil Jowell and his wife Kate are all smiles at the Mount Nelson Hotel after yesterday's lunch and presentation.'

At the time, quite apart from her obvious delight at Neil's success, there was much about which Kate could be pleased. Her career at the Business School continued to gain momentum. In 1987 she was nominated by the University of Cape Town's Commerce Faculty as its Distinguished Woman on the occasion of the university's Centenary of Women. Her role as senior lecturer had expanded to that of director of the Shell Industrial Relations Case Writing Institute at the Business School.

Then, in 1990, she was appointed associate professor, and in that year she also won the Business School's award for Most Outstanding Lecturer on the MBA 1989–90 Programme. Kate's influence outside academia continued to broaden: she was a member of the executive council of the Cape Chamber of Industries; she sat on the council of St Cyprian's School; she was honorary president of the South African Women's Squash Racket Association (even though she didn't actually play the game!), and a panel member of the Independent Mediation Service of South Africa (IMSSA).

Throughout this period, Kate was gaining a reputation for her mediation skills. A female client, who had engaged her to mediate in a 'seemingly intractable' property dispute, told journalist Zelda Gordon-Fish that, though 'rather humourless', Kate Jowell was 'incredibly disciplined and obviously a woman with very clear goals'.[304]

The client's first meeting with Kate had taken place at Glencoe Road. It was interrupted halfway when one of Kate's daughters arrived home unexpectedly early from school. The client relates the incident as follows: 'The child was very upset; she'd just learnt that her best friend had been killed in a motor-car accident. Kate excused herself and spent some time with her daughter. When she returned, she gave no long explanations; she just said, "Sorry about the break," and simply picked up where we'd left off.'

While Kate's action may have been open to a range of interpretations, her client didn't interpret it negatively. 'It's not that she didn't care; it's just that she is so very professional.'[305] The private Kate would not have confided in her client, even though she was also a woman and may even have had children of her own. She focused instead on the job at hand, offering her professional skills and keeping separate her personal concerns and her emotional reactions to an upsetting domestic situation.

In the light of this incident, it is easy to understand the client's comment: 'Kate Jowell strikes me as someone who's invented herself.' For, as the woman went on to tell Gordon-Fish, Kate was well packaged. She had, indeed, ensured that the image she presented to the professional world was impeccable.

But when Gordon-Fish put the comment to Kate and asked her to interpret that 'invent' in the context of her life, Kate was taken aback and 'fumbled for words'. Kate's response is revealing: 'It seems to suggest that I had some sort of plan. Maybe because if someone says to you, "I want to do more – I can do that," they would interpret it in this way, I think I've never been scared to take things on, I've made my own niche in various places and if that means "invent", well so be it.'[306]

There is a touching naivety in Kate's uncharacteristically inarticulate response, a charming unworldliness in this woman of the world who operated with such aplomb in a tough and exacting male domain.

Gordon-Fish went on to question whether Kate had paid a personal price for the respect and admiration that she had won from men. Her immediate response was to deny this, but on further reflection, she admitted that she had always been so busy that she didn't have time to see her close women friends. She confessed, in a rare moment of openness, 'I don't see myself like this. I sometimes feel inadequate – I feel my skills as a woman aren't that well honed.' It is tempting to ask what Kate meant by 'skills as a woman'. Did these relate to the nurturing role of mother, the supportive role of wife?

But the journalist did not probe further, so a definite answer eludes us. Instead, Gordon-Fish pursued a somewhat safer line of questioning: How, then, did women respond to her success? 'I don't pick up any animosity,' was Kate's tentative response – but she immediately changed tack. 'Well, maybe …' She then related an incident involving a discussion with a group of women parents regarding the school lift club. Kate was explaining the difficulty of fully participating because of her tight working schedule, when one of the women 'spat angrily': 'Why should I help you do what I would like to do myself?'

'I registered that,' Kate told Gordon-Fish, 'and decided if I ever needed anyone, it would have to be on a strictly quid pro quo basis.' Gordon-Fish's interpretation was that Kate Jowell never retreated from that decision, and never again asked for favours.[307]

She was right.

14

Down to Business

(1990–93)

O CTOBER 2003. I arrive at Glencoe Road to find Kate pacing up and down the top floor of the house. Her feet clatter rhythmically on the tiled floors, the sound changing only when she comes up against something that obscures her path. Then she paces on the spot until someone helps her around the obstacle. Increasingly, her gait is lopsided. No one – including her doctor – seems to know why.

I greet her, and she responds with a cheerful 'Hello', but her eyes are dull. 'Why are you here?' she asks, startling me. It's the first time that she has seemed confused by my appearance at the house. 'I'm here to take you to Carlucci's for a cappuccino, and to talk to you about the book,' I say, willing her to make the connection. But Kate remains silent, unresponsive.

For a few seconds she paces on the spot, then moves off, like a restless filly, skittish and troubled. Eunice explains, 'Mrs Jowell is not good today.' Eunice is sombre, and appears depressed.

Her world, and that of Kate Jowell, intersected for the first time in 1990. Their association and subsequent relationship was at once simple and complex, detached and intimate, a relationship governed by their roles – Kate the exacting employer, Eunice the efficient employee. On first meeting, neither woman could possibly have predicted how profoundly each would influence and affect the other's life in the years ahead.

Eunice is younger than Kate by a decade. A warm, wise, salt-of-the-earth character, she could, I imagine, be fierce if crossed or betrayed. Since I have been working with Kate, Eunice has often taken me into her confidence as she grapples with a metamorphosis she has not chosen, her role changing from housekeeper to caregiver, with all the in-between nuances. But she is much more than a mere caregiver – she is a constant companion, a confidante, managing the day of her once-powerful and independent employer with humour, restraint, humility and empathy. I have been struck on several occasions by Eunice's courage and resilience in dealing with a difficult, debilitating and, often, depressing situation.

Eunice's ability to handle Kate's decline, together with the advice, supervision and meticulous care provided by social worker Lindy Smit, has allowed the family to put off having to employ a full-time nurse/companion for Kate, who would almost certainly find this intrusive and traumatic, a constant reminder of the loss she has suffered on so many levels. As Justine remarked the first time I met her, 'Ma doesn't realise that Eunice is now her nurse.'

The unique curse of Alzheimer's, says David Shenk, is that it ravages several victims for every brain it infects.[308] First in line are loved ones and close friends, who are forced not only to witness 'an excruciating fade', but to also step in and compensate for the everyday abilities the person has lost as the brain slowly shuts down.

We all rely on other people in order to live full, rich lives. A person with dementia relies increasingly – and, in the fullness of time, *completely* – on the care of others, Shenk notes. 'The caregiver must preside over the degeneration of someone he or she loves very much; must do this for years and years with the news always getting worse, not better; must every few months learn to compensate for new shortcomings with makeshift remedies; must negotiate impossible requests and fantastic observations; must put up sometimes with deranged but at the same time very personal insults; and must somehow learn to smile through it all.'

Even for Eunice, looking after Kate is a relentless, daunting and, ultimately, thankless task. She has had to become adept at reading her once eloquent employer in order to diagnose a slew of ordinary and extraordinary ailments, from hunger to headaches, that Kate is unable to understand herself, let alone communicate to others.

The stress facing caregivers, notes Shenk, is so extraordinary that it often leads to very serious problems, including fatigue and forgetfulness, and these and other symptoms have aptly been described with the tongue-in-cheek term 'caregiver's dementia'. But there is nothing funny about this stress-induced psychological condition, and it is estimated that roughly half of all Alzheimer's caregivers struggle with clinical depression.

In the book *Alzheimer's Disease*, William Molloy and Paul Caldwell say that, apart from depression, caregivers also feel angry, frustrated and, above all, trapped. 'They feel inadequate – they feel they are not doing enough, caring enough, loving enough. The pressing needs are like a bottomless pit.'[309]

Then there's the loneliness. Caring for Kate at home, as Eunice does, is isolating, and the existence, for Kate as much as for her caregivers, is an insular one, says Lindy Smit.[310]

Lindy, who has been a regular at Glencoe Road since meeting Kate in 2002, stops by most Fridays. Her visits have become a lifeline, not only for Kate, but for Eunice too. Lindy has helped Eunice understand and manage not only Kate's illness but also her challenging role as a competent and compassionate caregiver.

There is no doubt the disease has affected Eunice profoundly. For, as doctors Molloy and Caldwell note, Alzheimer's spares no one. It creates victims and survivors, and caregivers need to care for themselves first and foremost. 'It's not selfish – it's survival. If you don't take care of yourself, the disease will kill both of you.'[311]

Yet always, whether she is having a good day or not, Eunice is pleased to see me. Today, however, instead of talking about how Kate is getting along, we talk about her own life – her childhood, her family, her relationship with 'Mrs Jowell'.

'When I first met Mrs Jowell, she was a very difficult lady,' Eunice says earnestly.[312] Reflecting on her choice of adjective, she explains that Kate liked things to be done 'properly'. 'She was very fussy, but once I got to know her ways, and her personality, it was fine.' Kate was particular about food: how it should be prepared and what time it should be served. For dinner at Glencoe Road, Eunice made 'things like stews, roast chicken, salad. Things like that.' And every night there was a routine dessert, to which Neil was especially partial.

Eunice was born in Dutywa, a small town in the Transkei. Her childhood was anything but happy. She and her only sibling, her brother Sicelo, were orphaned when their mother and father died within a year of one another. 'I was fourteen when my mother died,' Eunice tells me, 'and fifteen when we lost my father.' Her uncle, her mother's brother, stepped in to care for his niece and nephew, but the situation was far from ideal. 'He was nice to me, but his wife was not,' Eunice explains.

Eunice grew up in Dutywa, where she eventually married. She had two children, Yandisa and Xolile, who are now grown up, before the marriage ended. She never remarried, but had three other children with another partner: Nolundiso, Yoliswa and Vuyokazi (Vuvu), now also adults.

'When my children were growing up, I was a very strict mother,' she says with a grin. 'But I was also a friend to my children. They are not scared of me, but they know that I believe that things must be done properly. In that way, I am an old-fashioned mother.' She looks at me, eyes twinkling, then bursts out laughing.

Eunice migrated to Cape Town, all five children in tow, when she was thirty. She came, like thousands before and after her, to look for work. Her first job was with a Jewish family in Sea Point, and it was while she was in their employ that she read an advertisement in the smalls placed by Kate Jowell. Eunice got the job as housekeeper and cook.

Nicola was fourteen at the time; Justine was sixteen. Eunice provides an impromptu character sketch of the girls: Justine was 'a very, very nice girl, very friendly, with a soft heart'. Nicola was 'a bit shy', with a lovely smile. The girls were attached to their mother, Eunice notes. 'But it was difficult for them, because she travelled so much. But when she was home, you could see how close they were to her. She spoilt them at the weekends, taking them out, buying them things.'

Turning her thoughts to her employer's parenting of her girls, Eunice offers the insight that, in her view, Kate was a good mother who never raised her voice in anger. 'I never heard her shouting at them. She got on very well with her children. They loved and respected her. It was not her way to fight with them in front of other people. If she was annoyed, she'd call them into the study and talk to them.'[313]

About five years after becoming part of the Jowell household, Eunice noticed that Mrs Jowell's behaviour had begun to change. Her previously even-tempered, pleasant and charming employer was suddenly prone to mood swings and temper tantrums. 'I had never known her to be like that. I was sometimes afraid to approach her.'

Eunice recounts one of those days, when Kate was waiting for a driver to fetch her (she was still driving her own car at that stage) but there was some delay. She flew into a rage and kicked over a stack of Tupperware containers piled on the kitchen floor. She later apologised, but the outburst shocked Eunice, and scared her too. Kate had also become very forgetful. 'One day she flew to Johannesburg for a business meeting, and she forgot her jacket on the plane. And often, if she was going to the office, she would leave something behind,' Eunice says.[314]

~

For a long time now, Kate has stopped mentioning her affliction to me. And I, in turn, have become hesitant to refer to it. I wonder if she is delusional or in denial, or if she has truly forgotten that she is ill. When I first started speaking to her about her life and how it had come to this – to her 'rattling around' in a big house, almost always alone during the day apart from the company of Eunice – Kate would speak then, often casually, about being afflicted with Alzheimer's.

One morning she spontaneously announced, 'I was sitting in this house for years and finally I said to Neil, "Why am I sitting in the house on my own every day of the week?" Suddenly the penny dropped. And that's when Ivan appeared, to take me for a drive each week.' Her first outing with Ivan Jacobus, she recalled at the time, was to a screening of

Iris, the award-winning film on the life and death of the writer and philosopher Dame Iris Murdoch, herself a victim of Alzheimer's.

'I think someone tried to persuade me not to go,' Kate said earnestly. The person in question was Lindy. 'She said, "Perhaps it's not a good idea for you to see the film," and I said, "But this is what I've got, and I'm not going to try to disguise it."'[315]

I was hesitant to ask her what she'd made of the film, the story of the decline of an independent and fiercely intelligent woman into a state of child-like bewilderment, with the *Teletubbies* toddlers television programme a source of comfort and distraction. I sensed, as Kate recounted this incident, that she was beyond comprehending the horror of what lay ahead; how she – like Iris Murdoch, who had also once earned her living and built and sustained an identity from working with words – had ended up losing her ability to write or read them.

Kate's mind was already muddled and confused. The same day that she revealed her thoughts on Iris Murdoch, she told me about the problems she had taking her Alzheimer's medication. 'This morning I was putting my pills …' she began and then faltered. 'A pill this size,' she began again. 'I have Alzheimer's, and if I drop this pill it will be difficult for me to find it in this big house.' She'd just recounted what she called a 'spectacular' fight with Eunice about the pink pill, 'this tiny little pill'.[316] Eunice confirms Kate's account – that it is still a battle to get her to take the medication.

Initially, Kate got 'very upset and depressed' when the symptoms of her Alzheimer's began to become very evident.[317] When climbing the stairs, writing a note, making a cup of tea, when these mundane things became a struggle, Kate finally understood that her life would never be the same again.

I am haunted by whether she was able to reveal her feelings when she was grappling with the terrifying notion of losing her mind. How did she cope with the pain and the horror of realising that her brain was shutting down? I put the question to Nicola when she was in Cape Town on a visit. But it's a question she cannot answer. Kate didn't share her distress with her children. 'We've never had the ability to talk to our parents about those things,' Nicola says carefully. Kate would remark that she 'felt stupid' if a simple task became impossible for her to complete, but she never verbalised her fears. 'I imagine there was a long time when she felt very scared, and it's a great loss that we have not spoken about it,' Nicola says.

When I ask Neil, his eyes cloud over. 'She once broke down and cried, as she realised she might not see the girls married nor meet and enjoy her grandchildren. For the rest, she didn't really show the pain and suffering she must have felt.'[318]

Kate's increasing inability to negotiate her way up or down a flight of stairs was one of the first ways Alzheimer's curtailed her life and broke her spirit. Even in the year prior to our meeting, Kate's outings to the cinema, theatre and concerts – she was a regular at the Cape Town Concert Series of classical music performances – were becoming stressful. She became easily disorientated in surroundings that had previously been all too familiar.

Nicola tells how her mother, who was attending a concert on her own at the Baxter Theatre in Rondebosch one evening, left her seat at interval. When she returned to the auditorium for the second half of the performance, she sat in the wrong seat. 'She had to be pointed to the right place, as she didn't know where she had been sitting or how to find the seat. When she finally sat down in her original seat, the man sitting next to her remarked, "I hope you're not driving tonight …" He mistook her faltering movements and difficulty in finding her place for her having had too much to drink.' Her mother was 'very upset', Nicola says. 'That man was implying that she was drunk … but she has Alzheimer's. It's terribly sad.'[319]

There is a poignant irony in Nicola and Justine's disclosure that as young girls they had often implored their mother not to 'embarrass' them – Kate was often asked to speak at functions at their school, and they would do their best to discourage her. 'The funny thing is that once I'd matriculated, she did speak at a prize-giving function, and I happened to be in the audience. She was so good, and so funny. She began by telling everyone that one of her daughters was in the audience, hoping that she was not going to embarrass her!' Nicola went away from the function feeling very proud of Kate. It is a pride that has persisted: 'So many people have always commented to me about how much my mom has achieved. I feel really good when they do.'[320]

~

After sixteen years at the University of Cape Town Graduate School of Business, Kate Jowell was appointed associate professor in 1990. She had witnessed vast changes during that time, working under key directors, including Meyer Feldberg, John Simpson and David Hall.

Perhaps the most colourful director was the one whom Kate *didn't* get to work with – Bob Boland. One of the founders of the Business School, Bob Boland resigned in 1977. He had been away from the Business School for some time prior to his resignation, training instead to be a medical doctor through an accelerated learning programme at Juárez University in Mexico. In the Business School's 1978 *Journal*, which Kate edited, she wrote, 'Hundreds of delegates to the school over the past ten years will remember Professor Boland's enthusiasm and brilliance as a teacher of Management Accounting and Finance.'

An institution that 'dared to tilt at windmills', the Business School was conceived in 1963 by the distinguished dean of the Faculty of Commerce, Professor William Hutt. His idea was to create a school that resembled the better business schools in the United States. It was to prove a particularly difficult task, and 'only a man with Hutt's personality and single-minded determination could have pulled it off'.[321]

His proposals were not welcomed by colleagues, who found the concept of profit-making 'alien and abhorrent' in an academic environment. 'It went without saying that teaching people how to make money was even worse.'[322] A year later, just before he retired, Hutt was rewarded for his controversial efforts when the university's senate and council agreed to an official, experimental year. Old Mutual donated R100 000 to establish the Old Mutual Chair of Business Administration, which led to the Graduate School of Business and the institution of an MBA degree.

But Hutt, impatient at the delay in officially setting up the Business School, had in fact already begun teaching the first class of seventeen part-time students in January 1964. Six of these seventeen hopefuls graduated with UCT's first MBA degrees in 1966.

Hutt's successor was Bob Boland, a man who would make his mark in an extraordinary way. Described as 'energetic' and 'highly intelligent', Boland became a driving force second to none. He befriended 'people who counted', set up an advisory committee, and secured buildings, equipment and other logistics for the Business School 'with a speed that left some of his colleagues breathless'.

University House, a sprawling former residence that was about to be demolished, was converted into a self-contained unit to house the Business School. Initially regarded as temporary accommodation, the freshly painted bungalows would, however, be home to the Business School for decades to come.

Boland gathered together a formidable teaching team, including three visiting overseas professors; he introduced to the university 'an extroverted style of teaching, the likes of which the campus had never seen'. But however vibrant and stimulating as a place of learning, the Business School was 'in a state of organised chaos'.[323] It was only when Boland left in 1972 and his successor, Meyer Feldberg, took over, that the Business School really came into its own.

Feldberg, who had been recruited by Boland and had graduated with academic honours from Columbia University's Business School, changed the style of the UCT Business School by tuning in to the needs of the marketplace, reinforcing links with international business and teaching communities, and refining the MBA programme. By the late 1970s, the majority of UCT MBA graduates were establishing themselves in top management positions both locally and abroad.

Feldberg also substantially increased the workload of MBA students. 'You'll have little time for reflection,' he warned new students regarding the intensive programme upon which they were about to embark. He provided them with the best teaching talent he could find, in South Africa and abroad, often looking to the Business School itself for candidates. 'We literally have to breed them ourselves,' he confided in an interview at the time.[324] One of his protégées was Kate Jowell.

Trevor Williams, a 'quintessential Englishman who had first come to Cape Town in 1969 to teach at UCT's then Department of Commerce, was one of the Business School's first visiting lecturers; he had met Kate at that time, and still maintains ties with her and Neil. In 1974, while he was heading the Institute for Futures Research at the University of Stellenbosch, he was invited to teach a course in Statistics Operation and Computers at the UCT Business School.

There, 'in its shack accommodation on the lower slopes of the Rondebosch campus', he encountered Kate Jowell. 'Later, introducing me to people,' he confides in an email exchange from England, 'Kate invariably said that we had found ourselves neglected by the Business School and, orphan-like, sought platonic solace in each other's company.' Williams doesn't recall sharing Kate's view at the time, however. Instead, he was 'revelling in the near-autonomy granted by the Business School's director/s, and it seems unlikely that a woman so self-assured, self-contained and socially adept would have felt discomforted'. [325]

Indeed, his first impression of Kate was that she was 'cool'. I sense he doesn't mean that she was hip, or that she was distant and aloof, although other people may fairly readily have attributed these traits to her. To Williams, the young Kate Jowell had – at least in public – 'the coolness of Grace Kelly'. It is an interesting analogy: two beautiful, accomplished young women who had found their princes. But in many respects the two women's lives were worlds apart. Only a decade separated them in age, but while Grace Kelly's briefly brilliant film career was nipped in the bud by her marrying into the House of Grimaldi, Kate's marriage to Neil Jowell in no way stunted her career ambitions. And, unlike Princess Grace, Kate was not to retreat into a life of pampered luxury after marriage, nor did she believe, as Her Serene Highness did, that 'women's natural role is to be a pillar of the family ... the emancipation of women has made them lose their mystery'.[326]

Kate would never succumb to a traditional woman's role. It is notable, nevertheless, that although she was emancipated and a 'non-aggressive feminist', she retained that element of 'mystery' throughout her life. The Kate Jowell whom Trevor Williams got to know in the 1970s knew what she wanted, and in her singular, unruffled way, she set about getting it.

Williams recalls an incident, the first time they lunched together, that typified her approach and her manner: Kate had ordered fish, and, finding it not to her liking, she sent it back, as she had recently suffered from a bout of food poisoning and was wary of eating food that was not fresh or properly cooked. 'I can think of several occasions, and several apparently sophisticated people, where the incident might have been embarrassing to guest/s and/or the host,' Williams notes. But with Kate there was no such difficulty. She knew what she wanted – or in this case didn't want – 'and was entirely untroubled and untroubling in proceeding'.[327]

This 'Rondebosch fish non-incident', as Williams refers to it, was the first of many occasions over the years he has known her where Kate exhibited 'many "un" and "c" characteristics': she was untroubled, unruffled, unpretentious – and calm, courteous, considerate.

Like many other men who worked with her, Trevor Williams was not unaffected by Kate Jowell's style, warmth and graciousness. She may have been a feminist, but men were attracted rather than repelled by her intelligence and charmed by her natural ease. Williams goes on to state, somewhat tongue-in-cheek, 'of course there was more, on which a reticent Englishman could never comment' – then asks rhetorically whether at a restaurant in London in the late 1990s he may have been mistaken in detecting 'a spark of jealousy from the CEO of a related company as I, no doubt inconsiderately, sat down between him and Kate!'[328]

Kate took the attention of her male colleagues in her stride. Her book of cuttings contains an amusing hand-written note pertaining to her mediation skills, illustrating that she was not unaffected by the attention of powerful men. The note states, 'CMP has formed a union and has voted unanimously that if we *must* have an industrial relationship with anyone, we want to have an industrial relationship with *you*. The chapel has also asked me to sing a little song which goes like this: K-K-K Katie, beautiful Katie, You're the only girl the guys are asking for; When the workers strike over a pay rise, You can come and tell them why they can't have more.' The note was signed: 'With the compliments of the author Dan Curran, LTA Life.' Kate was yet to become a member of the IMSSA, but she was already well known – and obviously well liked – in industrial relations circles.

In the hallowed halls of academia, John Simpson, who succeeded Meyer Feldberg as Business School director in 1979, found Kate to be 'very discreet' but also 'distant'.[329] Yet his tenure as director, which stretched to 1986, was a crucial time for Kate. Simpson had helped her find her niche when she first joined the Business School, and his continued interest in the field of industrial relations would significantly shape her career path. Kate and Simpson eventually co-authored the groundbreaking *Cases in South African Business Management* (Juta & Company, Cape Town, 1979). Professor Simpson also appointed her as his assistant director, which caused tension among certain Business School academics – especially those who were better qualified and 'felt strongly that they should not have to report to her'.[330]

On the surface, Kate seemed to take it all in her stride and was 'fairly convivial' towards her colleagues, acknowledging their qualifications and understanding their position. But their attitude probably contributed to her determination to develop an area of expertise all her own, in spite of not having the academic qualifications to back it up.

The animosity of her colleagues aside, Kate's character, ambition and vision carried her through. 'She put a lot of effort into becoming an industrial relations expert at a time when there were very few people who were knowledgeable about the field,' Simpson recalls. [331]

As Business School director, John Simpson added 'depth and relevance' to the MBA programme and the school itself.[332] He was keen to establish the Business School as a seat of learning, encouraging lecturers to do research and publish academic papers, bringing in top overseas lecturers, upgrading the computer facilities and facilitating the creation of the Shell Industrial Relations Case Writing Institute. The Case Writing Institute, sponsored by Shell South Africa with a R200 000 donation over five years, was a huge breakthrough for the Business School. Created with the sole purpose of 'initiating, developing and disseminating appropriate case material on Industrial Relations and related matters for use ... by all participants in the labour debate', it provided the Business School with resources to develop an in-depth portfolio of relevant case studies and made the teaching of industrial relations unique and dynamic.[333]

The challenge for Kate, and colleagues such as Norman Faull, was developing and teaching an industrial relations course in the absence of textbooks and South African case material. Shell South Africa initially commissioned Faull – at the time a senior lecturer working on a doctoral thesis on the effect of industrial relations on productivity – to write up a seminal Volkswagen case, as it illustrated a range of principles.

Following the success of this venture, Shell South Africa sponsored the Case Writing Institute, and Kate was appointed its director. This provided, in her view, an opportunity to develop a portfolio of cases covering major aspects of South Africa's industrial relations in big companies. And the time was ripe for this. Kate commented that trade unions were challenging many aspects of management, and companies had to face issues of far broader concern than fair wages and grievance procedures.

'Business has to find ways of maximising the use of scarce resources, learn how to operate in an increasingly competitive global market, how to deal as good corporate citizens with the problem of massive unemployment, and recognise the need to upgrade skills of the workforce, given the increasingly acute shortage of such skills,' Kate noted in a special publication to celebrate the Business School's twenty-fifth year. 'It's vital that management and trade unions see these as joint problems that require a cooperative approach.'[334]

South Africa was, at the time, a country in a state of violent transition, and to meet the demands of the rapidly changing political, economic and social environment of the 1980s, Simpson reshaped the MBA programme. Not only was the Business School increasingly aware of its important role in a changing society, but UCT MBA graduates were also making their mark in the business world. A survey conducted in 1977 revealed that within ten years of the first MBA class graduating from UCT, over 25 per cent of students had become chairmen, managing directors and general managers of companies.[335]

By 1979, the figure had risen to 36 per cent, with a new survey showing that 70 per cent of all Business School graduates had clinched top or senior management positions. At the time, Simpson believed the Business School had a healthy future, as it was geared to meeting the 'coming changes in business and society'. But he also foresaw a problem that would become an increasingly pressing, and provocative, issue for tertiary education institutions in South Africa: he commented that it remained to be seen whether the challenge faced by the Business School might mean 'sacrificing standards to accommodate the students of our new society'. He hoped that certain bodies, including the Centre for African Management, created during his tenure, would 'help make the Business School more sensitive to the problems facing this country'.[336]

The Graduate School of Business would face its own set of problems, and the years following Simpson's tenure would prove more than challenging – both for its future directors and for the university itself. The appointment of Paul Sulcas as his successor proved highly controversial, and Sulcas faced a powerful lobby of disgruntled business academics, many of whom felt he was inexperienced and not the right person for the job.[337] True to form, Kate Jowell didn't join the fray, which by all accounts became 'petty', and most of her colleagues were therefore in the dark as to her opinions on Sulcas.[338] If indeed Kate ever did have a run-in with Sulcas, she would have considered it a private matter and no one would have been privy to it. Kate's characteristic discretion impressed former colleague Mike Page, who proved to be one of his former teacher's greatest allies.

Paul Sulcas presided over the Business School as it celebrated its twenty-fifth anniversary in October 1989. At a celebratory banquet in Cape Town, he paid tribute to his predecessors, especially Bob Boland, Meyer Feldberg and John Simpson, who had built the Business School into one of international repute. It was imperative, he felt, that it maintained its visible presence and standing in the marketplace.[339]

But while the Business School retained its reputation as an excellent place of learning, the internal squabbling among academics was 'filtering down into the student body', and the university authorities and the Commerce Faculty had become impatient and edgy with the state of affairs. At the end of 1989, two years after his appointment, Sulcas stepped down, and the position of director became vacant.

Kate Jowell applied for the job, and among the referees to back her bid for the director's chair she included her friend and Margo Commission colleague Jannie Graaff. In considering her suitability for the position, Graaff identified three key requirements he felt a Business School director should meet. The first was 'undoubted academic excellence', which would ensure she would be treated with respect; the second was 'a good personality ... someone who was well-liked'; and the third was a good business network to generate funds for the Business School.

'I thought that on those three things she did qualify,' Graaff says. The fact that Kate didn't have a doctorate 'worried' Graaff. But he brushed his concerns aside as one of his former fellow Cambridge students, who eventually went on to win the Nobel Prize in Physics, had become professor and head of the Physics Department at a leading United States university without ever having obtained a doctorate. 'With all this in mind, I decided that it didn't matter that Kate Jowell didn't have her PhD,' Graaff says.[340]

But the university was intent on appointing fresh blood, an academic of international standing, so David Hall, an outstanding scholar with a PhD from Harvard, was appointed director. Professor Hall had been briefly associated with the Business School as a visiting lecturer during the tenure of Bob Boland.

If the university authorities thought David Hall was going to still the troubled waters, they were wrong. Many Business School academics had the impression that Hall was given a mandate to 'get the idiots in line'.[341] This probably resulted in his not engaging his staff as he might have done, and instead of creating internal harmony, his single-minded approach resulted in continuing discontent. His staff were under the impression that he didn't value their contributions.

Mike Page, who on graduating with an MBA had himself joined the Business School as a lecturer in finance, concedes that the qualifications and publishing credentials of South Africa's business school academics probably 'falls short' by international standards. This is a somewhat spurious comparison to make, as South Africa's business school environment is, by nature of its geographical isolation, much smaller, and academics are deprived of ready access to the stimulation of international colleagues in their field. Nevertheless Page believes that 'when it comes to the ability of our academics to transfer their knowledge to executives and MBA students, they are right up there with the rest of the world – and that often gets overlooked. They have other strengths, and David Hall missed that.'[342]

David Hall will go down in the annals of Business School history for masterminding the school's move in January 1992 from its 'shack accommodation' in Rondebosch to the Breakwater Campus, with its prime real estate position at the Victoria & Alfred Waterfront. He had an agenda, and he pursued it vigorously, convincing the university authorities that the Business School could become a financially independent entity. However, the financial implications of the venture – or adventure, as some would have it – are still a point of contention, with some commentators noting that the Business School was not financially viable then, nor is it now.

Academically, the Business School falls under the Commerce Faculty, but as far as finances go, it reports directly to the vice-chancellor. Enjoying – and perhaps exploiting – its financially independent status, a them-and-us scenario came to prevail, and the Business School was frequently at loggerheads with the Commerce Faculty. The Business School's directors do not report directly to the Commerce Faculty dean, but rather to the vice-chancellor. John Simpson candidly admits that during his tenure as director he consciously worked at ensuring the Business School's independence from the Commerce Faculty. This was apparently David Hall's approach too, as he hatched an ambitious plan to move the Business School to its present location, 'pulling the wool over the eyes' of the powers-that-be.[343]

As Trevor Williams puts it, 'It's almost a matter of record that when David Hall became director, the move to the Breakwater Campus – and the financing of the Breakwater Lodge – happened, and it turned out that some people at the university were not very happy about what was going on.'[344] In certain respects, the move was a necessary one, as the Business School had long outgrown its shabby, cramped accommodation. Hall's ambitious plan to move to the other side of the city took the university authorities by surprise, and speculation has it that they agreed mainly because 'they didn't know what they were letting themselves in for'.[345]

The university agreed to Hall's plan on the proviso that the Business School be self-funding from the start. But the original funding to buy the building and meet the conditional interest payout fell short, and the university was forced to step in. This continued for the next five years.

Mike Page suggests that this should have come as no surprise to the authorities. 'You can't build a facility like that and not put any money into it. And even though the plan was far too ambitious, in the end the University of Cape Town got brilliant Business School premises.' But the reality of paying the tab 'startled' the university, and 'things got a bit tight between David Hall and the Commerce Faculty and Bremner [the building housing UCT's administrative offices]'.[346] The entire affair inevitably turned into a debacle, and David Hall, exhausted by the saga, left the Business School sooner than he expected to.

While Kate Jowell must have felt huge disappointment when her bid for the director's position failed, Hall's tenure turned out to augur well for her. He appointed her director of the MBA Programme – an important position at any business school – and she took up the challenge at a time when many perceived the Business School's image to be tarnished. 'David Hall was looking to jack up the Business School, and Kate had a great public profile,' observes Page.

Kate's reputation as a lecturer was confirmed when students awarded her the accolade 'Most Outstanding Lecturer on the MBA 1989–1990 Programme'. Her students saw her as a critical thinker who demanded much of them, and though they were all a little intimidated by her sharp intelligence, they liked and respected her.

She excelled as MBA programme director, and it is certainly due to her efforts and those of David Hall that the international reputation of the Business School was largely restored. This is borne out by the fact that, in 1992, more foreign MBA students registered at the University of Cape Town's Graduate School of Business than ever before. Of the eighty-six MBA students in 1992, twenty-two were non-South Africans. Foreign students clearly felt they could now study in South Africa as it was 'politically more respectable ... and a good thing to have on your CV, not a blot', as Kate explained in an interview with Gorry Bowes Taylor.

'We used to have foreigners on our MBA programme, but it got rather difficult in the late 1970s and early 1980s,' Kate noted.[347] At that time, a volatile political situation had prevailed in South Africa, characterised by unrest in black schools, in 1976 and again in 1980, and the academic boycott in 1984.[348] The revolt was against the apartheid system, but black pupils felt bitter and angry about the inferior standard of education they were receiving. The South African Institute of Race Relations revealed that, annually, the state was spending R1 385 on educating every white pupil, compared with R871 on every Indian pupil, R593 on every coloured pupil and R192 on every black pupil.

Government spending on black education increased dramatically under PW Botha's administration – from R68 million in 1978 to R237 million by mid-1985 – and by the early 1990s the political situation had stabilised to the extent where South Africa became attractive once more to foreign learners.

At the UCT Business School, David Hall was keen to see foreign students in his lecture rooms, and the Business School began an active campaign to target such students. Kate felt that foreign students added 'a valuable perspective to the classroom debate'.[349] She also believed that a particular attraction of the UCT MBA was the perception foreigners had of South Africa as an exciting country to visit, 'a place where a lot is happening and where there is a lot of opportunity'.[350]

The Business School's teaching methodology emphasised group learning. 'We put people into the classroom only after they've done a lot of reading and after they've talked about the reading and the assignments in small groups,' Kate explained. Only when students entered the classroom did they share their experiences, and the conclusions of their group, with the instructor facilitating the debate. 'It enriches the process to have people with a range of experiences, and it has been extremely stimulating having a big chunk of foreigners with their different cultural experiences. Some are a lot more assertive and aggressive than South Africans – which make for feisty debate,' she said.[351]

UCT's eleven-month MBA programme had a particularly tight schedule, and the Business School had the same number of contact hours (hours in the classroom) as many top overseas schools with a two-year programme. Discovering that several Ivy League schools had between 500 and 600 teaching hours, UCT rearranged its hours – effectively lengthening the study year, but shortening the study week – to give students more time to contemplate and absorb what they were learning.

'Some students say they can't believe they're going to survive the pace and get through all the work, but at the end of the first term find they've learnt more than they ever thought possible,' Kate told Gorry Bowes Taylor. But as she herself had discovered when she tackled her own MBA in the early 1970s, 'when you encourage a process of self-learning and provide a challenging environment, people rise to the challenge wonderfully'. And, like Kate herself, who had been a journalist when she enrolled in 1973, many of the foreign students came from a variety of disciplines rather than the predictable field of business or finance.

Looking down at a clutch of papers on her orderly desk, Kate said to Bowes Taylor that the breadth of students' expertise blew fresh air into the Business School and its MBA programme. 'Here's a neurosurgeon, a conservationist, a crocodile farmer, an inventor, a poet. That's the enriching and learning process. This course is about fun, not just about work. Many find it one of the best years of their lives.'

Kate Jowell was determined that her MBA programme would prove to be just that – fun. But for David Hall, there was trouble in paradise. His conflict with university authorities showed no signs of abating, and in 1993, a year after the Business School's move to the Breakwater Campus – which Kate described as an outstanding success – Hall left the University of Cape Town. The director's chair was vacant once more.

~

During these tumultuous, triumphant times at the Business School, Kate's private world was fragmented: her daughters were teenagers caught up in a flurry of school and social activity; Neil continued to maintain a busy schedule during the week and pursued his sporting passions – cycling and squash – at weekends; her brother was living in the United States; and her mother had moved back to Cape Town following the death of Kate's father.

Kate still worked long hours, and, once or twice, she and Neil met purely by chance at business functions where neither expected to encounter the other. As an influential and high-powered couple, they were often on the same guest lists. On 10 May 1990, they wrote to President FW de Klerk and his wife Marike, thanking the presidential pair for including them in a cocktail function: 'We would have very much enjoyed meeting you both on any occasion but the coincidence with the Groote Schuur Accord made the evening doubly memorable. It's taken thirty years for South Africa to turn its back on Sharpeville. Our congratulations to you for the courageous part you have played in that process and good wishes for the future.'

Kate used functions such as these to build her business network. She was, by her very nature, a meticulous person, intent on absorbing every detail of people, places and events, and storing these in a way that would prove useful to her in another context, time or place. Whenever she met someone interesting, she would record his or her details on a filing card. Of M Key, whom she met in 1989 when he was director of the Duros Group, she wrote: 'Sat next to him. This is the Shell that bought City Tramways/Tollgate. He was a lawyer in Johannesburg who got a consortium together with two others. Reserved about his background. Somewhat uninformed about Trencor's scope despite having involvement with United Transport in his background. Quite impressive overall.' Often she would note personal family details. 'Son at Bishops,' she wrote of one person. 'A rugby player ... his wife cooks for the Barclays lunches'.

At their dinner parties, the Jowells continued to offer guests a combination of excellent company, superb food and fine wines. Some guests were more influential than others, but all enjoyed Kate and Neil's charming, generous hospitality. One fascinating guest was Henry R Kravis, the New York financier, investor and art patron regarded as one of the most successful investment bankers in history, and listed by *Forbes* in 2004 as being worth $1.3 billion. Kravis, a partner of Kohlberg, Kravis, Roberts (KKR), is famous for pioneering the leveraged buyout (LBO) and, in particular, for his acquisition in the late 1980s of RJR Nabisco for $25 billion.[352]

Like Neil, Kravis was an MBA graduate of Columbia University. When he visited Cape Town, the Jowells invited him to dinner, and Kate included Mike Page and his wife Sue on the guest list. Mike was delighted – but also surprised. 'We're talking about people in a different financial league, and Kate could have invited a whole host of people, but she thought to herself, "It'll be nice for Mike to meet Kravis", and that's what's so amazing about her, that side of her is awesome,' Page notes.[353] And, he goes on to add, Kate held her own in 'company like that'.

Trevor Williams likewise commends the Jowells for being impeccable hosts. He recalls an incident the first time he dined at Glencoe Road, when Kate invited him to meet Neil. Towards the end of the evening,

Neil opened a fine bottle of red wine for Trevor. Then, the next morning, courtesy of Neil, Kate presented the remains of the almost-full bottle to Trevor at the Business School.

'It was an example of Neil's kindness and consideration, as he knew I had particularly enjoyed it.' For Williams, years later, the gesture remains 'a unique experience that extended beyond the evening'.[354]

Justine and Nicola were, by now, used to the peculiarities of their home life, and they handled the situation with grace and good humour, as a joint card they sent to their parents at the end of 1989 illustrates. They wrote (the words emboldened by a rough and enthusiastic attempt at calligraphy): 'This is to Certify that Neil and Kate are sane even after a significant period of intense strain suffered by all parents.'

The 'strain' they allude to is probably the normal challenges most parents of teenagers encounter, but the frenetic pace at which Justine and Nicola's parents operated, and the many demands placed on them, would certainly have imposed a unique kind of strain on their parents. After a long and hard working week, Kate and Neil didn't regroup for family time. They pursued different interests at weekends.

'In my late adolescence, my parents were both working so hard that I think they didn't see as much of one another as they would have liked,' Justine reminisces.[355] 'Ma, Justine and I would spend the weekends together,' Nicola confirms. 'We'd go shopping, or we'd go away to our house in Hermanus a couple of weekends during the year. Pa was always busy on Saturdays – often working in the morning and playing squash in the afternoon. On Sundays, he cycled.'[356]

Neil's interest in cycling was ignited in the early 1980s after an operation to remedy an old knee injury he'd sustained on the rugby field curtailed his squash-playing activities. 'The operation was very conservative, but it laid me low for three months,' Neil explains, sitting at his desk in his study during one of our evening chats at Glencoe Road. 'I worked very hard at getting back to normal, and I succeeded, and returned to the squash courts.'[357]

Occasional knee problems persisted. Then his squash partner, Ralph

Ginsberg, who had just started cycling, invited Neil to join him on a ride. Neil was intrigued. 'I asked him where he planned to ride to, and he said to Simon's Town ... and back,' Neil says.[358]

He had felt daunted by the distance at first, but nevertheless took on the challenge. Neil cycled the thirty-odd kilometres from Cape Town to Simon's Town, South Africa's naval base on the False Bay coast, and then back again on a bicycle Kate and the girls had bought for him in 1980 while they were in America.

'I thought I was Superman,' he says, laughing. 'I thought it was a tremendous achievement.' For a man in his fifties, it probably was something of an achievement. But while he was rather pleased with himself, he was not yet completely 'hooked' on the sport. That would only happen three years later.

'We had planned a weekend to Hermanus, and I was not that keen to go because I wanted to stay in Cape Town and cycle,' he explains. Kate suggested he take his bike to Hermanus, which gave him the idea of cycling to the seaside town on Walker Bay. 'We decided that I would start cycling a while before they were due to leave by car, and they would pick me up along the road.' Early one hot Friday afternoon, Neil was duly deposited in Somerset West with his bike. 'I got out of the car, looked up, and saw this mountain shimmering in the haze, and I thought to myself, "You must be mad! You won't get up Sir Lowry's Pass!" So I started cycling, fully expecting Kate and the girls to help me out of this predicament, but they didn't come, so I had to carry on cycling. Eventually, when I was about ten kilometres from Hermanus, they caught up with me. They couldn't believe how far I'd got, and it was this that got me cycling seriously!'[359]

Today Neil has two bicycles – a Peugeot and a Look. The latter, with its French frame and nice gadgetry, is, as he says, 'quite a good bike'. 'It's beautifully designed – the wheels, the pedals and the handlebars are all aesthetically pleasing, functional and aligned.'

I ask Kate, who is sitting next to me, if Neil looks good when he goes cycling. 'I think so,' she says, with some hesitation. 'Does he have special gear?' I ask, trying to engage her in conversation. 'Yes,' she says, smiling, then falls silent, unsure of what to say next. 'Oh yes,' Neil interjects with a laugh. Cycling is a hobby he shares with his eldest son, David, who 'takes about half an hour to get dressed before he goes on a ride'. Neil smiles as he says, 'He has really nice cycling gear, and he gave me a smart jacket and glasses for my seventieth birthday.'

It's 9 p.m. by now, and Kate is shifting uncomfortably in her seat. Neil realises that she's exhausted, and excuses himself briefly to put her to bed and make her comfortable for what is probably going to be a long and restless night.

Alone in the study, I picture Neil cycling to Hermanus under the hot midday sun. The Jowells' Hermanus house is often on Kate's mind. When I first met her she mentioned it and gave me a rough account of how she used to manage their weekends there, the lists she had of what food to take along and when it was to be eaten. 'The house is in Kwaai-water. The last time I went there was with Ivan, but we couldn't get in because it was locked, and I had forgotten to take the house keys,' she said with a frown, as if she found the memory troubling.

The Jowells retreated to their Hermanus house, bought in 1985, at least three times a year, sometimes more. But as Kate's decline accelerated, what used to be a relaxing break became fraught and difficult. Their last visit, in Easter 2002, was not pleasant. 'I had to do all the cooking, something I'm not very good at,' Neil admits wryly, 'and Kate became very confused. She couldn't find her way around the house, couldn't find the toilet. To lose your way around a house you have known for nearly twenty years is very disconcerting and traumatic.'[360]

Since that time, they have never returned as a couple, or as a family, and their reluctant abandonment of a happy family ritual was surely another in a series of blows and a further sign that Alzheimer's disease was defeating not only Kate, and curtailing not only her life and her movements, but those of her family, too.

15

In the Director's Chair

(1993–99)

NOVEMBER 2003. The black road, slick with rain, bends in a wide
arc in the heart of Cape Town's Victoria & Alfred Waterfront.
Stately cranes, their symmetry etched against the grey sky, hover over a
multimillion-rand marina development under construction.

It's an unusually wet summer's day. Rain lashes my windscreen, and as
I round the corner, a squat white building with four turrets looms above
the roadway. Its elevation gives the site a commanding view of Table
Mountain – today shrouded in grey – and the marina across the way.

A metal sign flashes past. The lettering, in navy blue, reads simply:
The University of Cape Town – The Graduate School of Business. The
V&A Waterfront, one of the city's most popular destinations, is an
incongruous setting for the university's Breakwater Campus.

Thinking about this, I lean into the rain as I dash towards the doors
of the dumpy, two-storey building. Once inside, I'm surprised by its
modernity, expressed in unexpected architectural elements of glass
and steel. As I get my bearings, a student rushes in, a beanie protecting
his head from the cold. He greets a fellow student with a cheerful '*Molo!*
What's up?' as he casually puts his arm around her and leads her down
the corridor.

At one time, this was Kate Jowell's turf, and suddenly, in my mind's
eye, I see her striding purposefully down this corridor, wearing the
powder-blue blazer and determined smile captured in a photograph
over which I have often pored.

I set off to find the director's office, taking in the heavy steel doorways and gunmetal grey bars on the inner windows. At intervals, there are loudspeakers attached to the walls. These strange features are remnants of the building's past function as the old Breakwater Prison, a Cape Colony jail built in 1859 to house long-term convicts who'd been brought in to construct the breakwater in Table Bay. Later, in 1902, the Industrial Breakwater Prison, with its four castellated turrets, was erected to house 200 white prisoners, signalling the advent of separate institutions for black and white inmates. The design, with its turrets and enclosed courtyard, emulates that of Millbank and Pentonville prisons in England.[361] It was used as a convict station for only ten years, after which it housed juvenile offenders and, later, black dockworkers. Then, in the early 1990s, thanks to the ambitious plan conceived by David Hall, it became the troubled home of the Graduate School of Business.

The leather soles of my shoes loudly slap the metal staircase that leads to the director's office. The present incumbent is Professor Nick Segal, but I am especially interested in the room, because it is the same one Kate Jowell occupied when, on 1 February 1993, she became the first woman in South Africa to head a business school.

Her appointment was the pinnacle of her career, and the Business School gained a director who was not merely a good academic and networker, but also a vibrant personality with a national profile, married to one of the country's top businessmen.

In my mind's eye I had conjured up a roomy, impressive office that might somehow reflect the prestige and power of the position. In reality, though, it is a compact, modest space, its only defining feature the view from the double doors that lead onto a sliver of balcony.

The view is not of Table Mountain, as one would expect, but of the inner courtyard where prisoners presumably once took their daily exercise, and where students now stroll, scurry or sit.

I imagine Kate ensconced behind the desk, making decisions, meeting students. The rather ordinary floor-to-ceiling melamine bookshelves that cover one wall would certainly have bowed under the weight of her books. Given her keen aesthetic sense, there would have been original artworks on the walls, and fragrant blooms would have brightened her neat work space.

Kate Jowell had always shown the potential for occupying the position of director of UCT's Graduate School of Business. She certainly had the profile, and the presence, confirms Professor Norman Faull, who first met her in 1977 when she taught his MBA class.[362] She also had the ambition and the drive. Other colleagues who have known her for decades, like Professor Frank Horwitz (who would become the Business School's director in 2004), believe she had always aspired to the position.

On two occasions, Kate's attempts to realise her dream were thwarted. But she was not easily discouraged. 'From the time I met her in 1986, when she was assistant director to John Simpson, it was quite clear that she had an aspiration to become director,' says Horwitz.[363]

Norman Faull recalls Kate's bid for the position in 1987, when they were both persuaded to apply for the job. Neither of them succeeded, and Kate greeted the outcome with good humour, remarking that she felt as if she'd just missed being hit by a fast-moving train. Faull says she seemed relieved. But, with her ambitious nature, Kate must surely have felt regret, too. For she kept her eye on the position. After Kate had been promoted to associate professor under David Hall, her next logical career challenge was being appointed director of the Business School.

The opportunity arose when Hall resigned after two turbulent years in the director's chair. Kate was asked to fill his shoes as acting director, but she was not interested in doing so. 'Acting is not for you,' she told herself.[364] So instead, Frank Horwitz obliged.

The position of director was advertised nationally and also abroad – including in the prestigious British weekly *The Economist*. International business academics applied. Local hopefuls did the same. Kate was not among them. Perhaps she was simply too proud, having been overlooked when she first put her name forward. Or possibly she was fed up with the university for the way in which it had handled the situation. However, when the selection committee noticed the lack of strong internal candidates on its shortlist, Kate was asked her to apply – which she duly did.

Norman Faull, who was on the selection committee, says Kate's main competitor was an Australian academic with a passion for public administration. His vision that the Business School become involved in that arena alienated some members of the selection committee, including Faull and other Business School colleagues, who feared that the school would be hijacked. 'I came down on the side of Kate, and I can't say that she ever gave me cause to regret that decision,' Faull says.[365]

Kate was delighted with her appointment. She downplayed the fact that she had reached another first in her career as the first woman to head a South African business school: 'I've been one of the chaps for so long.'[366] Yet her unique flair and femininity would undoubtedly have added panache to the post.

Kate's appointment was well received. Cards, letters and faxes of congratulation streamed in from well-wishers, and these were eventually stored in a bulging file. She was proud of the Business School. She valued its international reputation, its ability to attract excellent candidates and academics. Her only regret about her new job was that she'd have less time with her students, the bright individuals she'd always loved teaching.[367]

But a daunting task lay ahead of her. Right from the start, it was an ominous challenge. Faull points out that the era she had to manage was 'horrible': 'There is,' he asserted, 'no other word for it.'

The Business School was in the process of reinventing itself. As director, Kate was, in effect, heading an academic school *and* a flailing business, inheriting the unenviable task of finding long-term backing for R40 million in medium-term debt.

Still smarting from David Hall's manoeuvre to house the Business School in a location it could not afford and would not be able to finance, vice-chancellor Stuart Saunders and the University Council sought a scapegoat.[368] Hall was the obvious victim, but with his departure, the new director came under fire. Says Faull, 'Hall had come up with a business plan that was not worth the paper it was written on, but the university went along with it. To pay for the building alone, the Business School would have to increase its revenue sixfold.'

When Kate accepted the position of director, she did so without preconditions. Faull believes this was a mistake. The most obvious precondition Kate should have insisted on was that the university take over the Business School's debt. 'I think Kate felt culpable in a certain sense because she had been a senior staff member under David Hall. The collective senior staff was held accountable for the fiasco.'

But, as Faull points out, if the university did not expect any of its other faculties to fund their own buildings, why should this be a requirement of its Business School?

Apart from her position as director of the Business School, Kate was also a director of the Graduate School of Business Company, a legal structure set up with the acquisition of the building. 'The university held Kate accountable for the debt, and they were terribly nasty to her,' Faull says.

Mike Page, Kate's close ally, believes the university appointed Kate to the job not only because she had the credentials, but because it believed she would be able to raise the necessary funding the Business School urgently needed. However, as Page points out, this was not Kate's style: 'Had they known her at all, they would have realised that it was not her way. She would never lean on people for favours.'[369]

Even so, right from the start Kate placed great emphasis on sustaining and expanding the Business School's links with the greater business and political community. She reaffirmed the Business School's mission statement, namely 'to contribute to the economic and social growth of southern Africa ... through developmental and research programmes aimed at enhancing the vision, the judgment and the effectiveness of managers and potential managers in all organisational settings'.[370]

Kate was intent on getting the Business School back on track: she pursued a standard of excellence, and urged her colleagues to produce papers that were of a high standard. In addition, she was keen to rebuild the shattered internal harmony, albeit subtly. She encouraged academics to pursue their interests and gave them the necessary space to do so. Once they succeeded, she recognised their contributions. Many of her colleagues, including Mike Page, believe she allowed the senior faculty to determine the direction of the school, such was her faith in her teaching staff.

Ever the perfectionist, Kate gave '500 per cent of her time' and expected the same level of commitment from those around her.[371] To some, she was a workaholic and a demanding taskmaster. She reacted to incompetence with coolness. Once, on hearing that a lecturer was not coping with the task and frustrating students with his lack of skills, she quietly entered the lecture room during one of his sessions to judge the situation for herself. The lecturer, who was already uncomfortable and out of his depth, blanched at the sight of Kate.

'He was clearly panicking,' reports a student. 'He was sweating profusely. We started to feel sorry for him, but Kate just sat there, quietly, watching him fall apart.' Clearly, she was not going to let him off the hook. Or at least that was the impression she gave. Shortly after this incident, his lecture series came to an end, so it's unclear whether she had acted on the situation or not.

Kate's aloofness was felt by many. 'She was very formal with people,' says Frank Horwitz. 'She was cordial and professional with her staff and her students.' Even her relationship with her personal assistant, Yvonne van Stolk, was not particularly close. Yet Kate commanded loyalty from her staff. 'Even though she seemed distant because she was so focused on her work, she really gave her heart and soul to the job. We knew how much she put in,' Van Stolk observes.[372]

While the demands of the job seem to have robbed Kate of a certain *joie de vivre*, colleagues and students sensed another side to her. They were struck by Kate's kindness. She was empathetic, and made time for people who needed help or a sympathetic ear.

Frank Horwitz, currently director of Cranfield School of Management, Cranfield University in Bedfordshire in the United Kingdom, says she was very supportive in small but crucial ways. If one of her staff gave a public lecture that was well received, Kate would send the lecturer a complimentary note. If her staff received good teaching evaluations, she responded by congratulating them. These gestures were appreciated, says Horwitz, who did not himself have a close relationship with Kate, however.[373] While they never collaborated, they did work well together.

Students also held her in high regard. In a light-hearted internal publication, the *Screaming Organ*, the MBA Class of '94 referred to her as 'our gracious and fearsome leader'. In a humorous mini-profile of their director, they wrote of her nocturnal prowling of the Breakwater corridors, working morning, noon and night, attending scores of functions and sending emails at all hours. On top of this, she was married to the chairman of a major South African company and was managing to raise two teenage daughters. Their director was someone who 'dots the i's and crosses the t's of every memo, letter and message that crosses her desk, and still manages to maintain a perfectly groomed image'. Tongue firmly in cheek, the students attributed Kate's 'mild obsessive compulsive behaviour' to her convent education!

Beyond the enigma, though, the students saw a Kate whom they described in their rough guide as expressing amusement by laughing; annoyance by drawing her eyebrows together and pursing her lips; surprise by lifting her eyebrows or inhaling 'sharply across clenched teeth' – when she was frustrated she exhaled 'sharply through a partially open mouth'; stress by brushing her hair from her face or putting it behind her ears; sympathy by 'maintaining concerted eye contact while you explain'; and concentration by talking 'while looking at nothing in particular'. For relaxation, they mused, 'Kate does nothing, she has no time, although she does pound the pavements of Higgovale in the early morning and go to gym sometimes.'

Kate must surely have smiled at this character sketch and its accompanying cartoon that exaggerated her black bob, spectacles and graceful neck.

Yet fun was probably the last thing on her mind during the turbulent

1990s. Politically, South Africa was tense and at times unstable. In a bid to defuse the situation and put South Africa on the road to reform, President FW de Klerk opened Parliament on 2 February 1990 with a historic address that stunned South Africa and the world: he unbanned thirty-four organisations, including the African National Congress. This was followed, on 11 February, by the release of Nelson Mandela after nearly three decades behind bars.

The nation was jubilant. Large-scale reform was on the cards, and the process of forging a new post-apartheid constitution had begun. But complex issues remained unresolved. On 17 June 1992, a gang of 200 men armed with guns and pangas attacked the Boipatong informal settlement near Johannesburg. Thirty-nine people died. Many more were injured. The next year, on 10 April, this massacre was followed by the assassination of Chris Hani, the charismatic leader of the South African Communist Party, who was gunned down outside his home in Boksburg, just outside Johannesburg.

It was a quiet Sunday morning. The former commander of the ANC's armed wing, Umkhonto we Sizwe (MK), was returning home from his local shop with the Sunday newspapers when a hail of bullets ended his life.

The murder was shocking; turmoil ensued. The political negotiations at the Congress for a Democratic South Africa (Codesa) were suspended, the foreign exchange rate and the share market slumped, and there were violent protests in Cape Town, Port Elizabeth, Durban and Pietermaritzburg.[374] Nelson Mandela appealed for calm. Fortunately, discussions on the future of the nation resumed, and a month later the Negotiating Forum announced the date of the first democratic election: 27 April 1994.

At the University of Cape Town, moves were already afoot to make tertiary education more accessible to students previously excluded for either academic or financial reasons. In one of her first interviews as director of the Graduate School of Business, Kate insisted that its aim was to turn out well-rounded managers – of whatever race or gender – who were equipped with the skills needed in South Africa's current environment. She conceded that a major recruitment drive was needed to enlist more women, as well as black and coloured students.[375]

Kate recognised the need for the university – and its Business School – to widen its reach in terms of the racial make-up of its student body. Yet she dismissed as nonsensical the notion that the Business School should in the process lower admission standards for its prestigious MBA course. Kate was inflexible on the matter: 'We are known for our product and we have to go on producing it.'[376]

Candidates for the course had always been screened and selected with care. Those who made the grade were all expected to pass. 'Our students,' she said, 'have an average age of thirty-two and we aim at a particular level of academic achievement, and people with the motivation to succeed.' She pointed out that the Business School was already producing black managers, and she predicted that the two black students who had graduated in 1992 would do exceptionally well. 'We don't see it as our task to change our MBA profile. We believe we have an obligation to ensure the development of managers in this country – but that does not mean that we have to take everyone,' she reiterated.

Regarding the paucity of female candidates, Kate surmised that women were either hesitant or reluctant to attempt an MBA because they lacked confidence. 'Research shows that successful professional women often have a successful man in the background – it could be a husband or a father – who believes in them and does not make them feel threatened as women if they succeed.'[377]

Kate herself continued to blaze a trail for career women. In 1993, the same year she was elected to head UCT's Business School, she also became the first woman appointed to the board of directors of Afrikaans insurance giant Sanlam, an astonishing feat for a British immigrant with a shaky grasp of the Afrikaans language. But Sanlam had chosen wisely: Kate was a conscientious board member, having already proved her mettle at First National Bank, where she'd been on the Western Cape board for years. A board appointment at Cadbury Schweppes soon followed.

Yet in spite of other commitments, her focus remained resolutely on the Business School, and she was intent on making it the top school in Africa. 'It's not just a wish, it's a passion,' she asserted.[378] Her interest was not merely professional. She herself held an MBA from UCT, and had a vested interest in protecting the qualification. 'I am a bearer of that currency,' she said, 'and I, like all our alumni, want to see that my investment in my MBA is protected by continuing high standards.'[379]

Kate's efforts were rewarded when, in 1995, the Business School was rated South Africa's top business school in a survey undertaken by *Professional Management Review* and conducted among 100 randomly chosen human resource directors of the top 300 companies in the country. Respondents were asked to rate fourteen institutions, and UCT beat its rival, the University of the Witwatersrand (Wits), by a narrow margin. Kate was delighted – it had been a competitive year with at least half a dozen US, UK and Australian business schools of varying levels targeting the business education market in South Africa.[380] In Kate's view, UCT's ranking positioned South Africa's traditional business schools way ahead of foreign distance-learning institutions.

Two years later, in 1997, the *Review*'s results confirmed Kate's opinion when its survey indicated that South African businesses continued to prefer local business schools over the rash of newcomers boasting international accreditation. This time round, UCT shared top position with Wits, scoring 8.11 out of a possible 10. But Kate must surely have been disappointed that Wits was voted most admired business school that year, and that big business saw it as a leader in its field. The survey also showed that Wits graduates were the most sought-after, followed by those from Unisa's Graduate School of Business Leadership and, in third place, those from UCT.

Kate remained undaunted, however. Four years into her term, 1997 was to prove a bumper year for UCT: the Business School was preparing for its largest ever full-time and part-time classes, with scores of black students having registered. In an interview with the *Sunday Times*, Kate revealed that there had also been a steady rise in the GMAT score – an internationally recognised admission test for MBAs.[381] By this time,

Mike Page was working closely with Kate as director of the MBA Programme. He told the *Sunday Times* that UCT's Business School was the only South African school that required candidates to pass the GMAT. 'We still strive for a balanced class in terms of work experience, maturity, academic ability and diversity,' Kate elaborated.

Like other South African institutions, UCT was embarking on a difficult and painful transformation process.

Ironically, Kate's relationship with Bremner – already strained owing to the financial predicament of the Business School – deteriorated further when another formidable woman became head of the University of Cape Town. Early in 1997, Dr Mamphela Ramphele succeeded Dr Stuart Saunders as UCT's vice-chancellor, becoming the first black woman to hold this office at a South African university. A qualified medical doctor with a string of degrees to her name, Dr Ramphele is a strong personality who manages with ease, confidence and style in a man's world. Extremely well connected, she has been involved in social upliftment most of her adult life.

Ramphele was not new to UCT. She had been a deputy vice-chancellor for five years prior to becoming vice-chancellor. And she'd been closely involved in developing an equity framework that focused on access, individual development and transformation. Her vision for South Africa's oldest tertiary education institution was that it should evolve into a world-class African university – without losing its reputation as a respected place of learning.[382]

But for all this, right from the beginning, Kate found a foe, not a friend, in Ramphele. It is difficult to pinpoint the exact reasons for their chilly relationship, but it is widely acknowledged. 'It was very difficult to understand their relationship,' Frank Horwitz confides.[383] It's possible they clashed because they were both high-achieving individuals, he offers. This may have been a factor, but, as Horwitz suggests, it was not the primary factor. 'Mamphela Ramphele was well connected in circles outside the university, which, perhaps, did not support Kate's appointment as director.'[384]

Another possible factor in the icy relationship that developed was Kate's steely resolve to maintain the exceptionally high standard of the Business School's MBA.

'Ramphele was keen to reform the university and saw the Business School as an elite institution,' says Bob Rotberg,[385] an acquaintance of both women. 'Kate, on the other hand, was trying to retain the Business School's special character. It's possible that the conflict was about how Kate ran the school,' Rotberg speculates.[386]

Neil Jowell puts it down to Ramphele's opposing Kate's appointment to the national board of directors of First National Bank. 'Kate sought the advice of Ian Simms, who was chairman of the university council at the time, because she couldn't see any reason as to why she should not accept the directorship,' Neil says.[387] Kate went ahead and the matter was never resolved.

In her day, Kate would have matched many of Ramphele's characteristics: both were strong, ambitious women – talented, outspoken, influential. Kate didn't have the political credentials – she was by nature not an activist, as Albie Sachs had discovered to his chagrin – but she had been at the forefront of labour reform for years, and was also a voluble critic of apartheid and the government. Perhaps, ironically, the differences between the two women stemmed from their similarities.

Kate saw her job essentially as one that involved people – students, academics, the business community – and identifying their needs was paramount.[388] She wanted to unearth talent, to nurture it, to equip people with the skills they needed and the space in which to use them.

She had worked closely with David Hall to establish the Associate in Management (AIM) programme – a nine-month intensive residential course for which no educational qualifications were required. It was, fundamentally, an affirmative action programme for students who needed intensive education at junior management level. In a radio interview, Kate admitted that white males dominated most of the Business School's programmes. 'But at junior level, there is a preponderance of black people, and a large number of women, and we are targeting that niche,' she added. The aim was to equip these students with the skills and confidence they needed to return to the workplace and thrive.

Kate's goals were clear: 'We give people the education they need, but also the negotiating, communication, numeracy and literacy skills, so that they're able to convey plans and ideas, and generally be more effective in their work environment.'

Teaching students *how* to learn had always been the Business School's approach. Diversity and different perspectives were crucial to the learning process. 'There is nothing more potent than having a group of five people assigned to work together, and among them, like we have this year, are an MK brigadier, two Chinese students from Beijing, a forester with twenty-two years' experience and a social worker who needs management skills,' she explained. 'Put these people together, and they learn a tremendous amount simply because they bring different perspectives to the same problem.'[389] Of course, history had precluded most South Africans from this sharing process, but Kate threw herself into the task of encouraging the sharing of common interests and goals – and differences as well – and mediating these in an educational environment.

Kate drew top individuals to the Business School, the benefits of which were certainly felt by her students. Professor John Simpson notes her wide range of contacts that enabled her to invite presidents – FW de Klerk and his then wife Marike once visited the school – and politicians to address the Business School.[390]

In analysing her contribution, Simpson credits Kate with doing a good job, especially considering the constraints under which she worked. 'I am absolutely sure she was a great success in getting recognition from the business community and government – that was her strength – and I am sure she procured funding, which the school needed desperately at the time.'[391]

~

November 2003. I watch idly as the wind whips the foamy tips off the waves as they rush towards the Mouille Point shore. There is a comfortable hum inside the snug seafront deli-café where I'm contemplating the life of Kate Jowell. Just down the road is the V&A Waterfront, and Kate's old stomping ground, the Breakwater Campus. I think about Kate the woman, Kate the wife, Kate the 'non-aggressive feminist', as Trevor Williams described her.

Mostly, though, I think about Kate the mother. In many of my conversations with people who have known or have come into contact with Kate and her daughters over the years, a constant refrain has emerged about how lovely they are, Justine and Nicola, and what a wonderful job Kate has done raising them. It is almost as if, frustrated by Kate's inscrutability, her intensely private nature, these people have been pleasantly surprised by her unassuming, gracious daughters. In Justine and Nicola, a side of Kate is revealed that very few people ever get to see.

I mull over this impression of Kate's success as a mother as I leave the seaside café and drive to Glencoe Road. Like any other working mother, Kate lived in the hope that she had done a decent job. In a radio interview in 1993 she revealed that her daughters were used to her pressurised programme: 'Luckily they are very independent, because I have worked ever since they were born.' She described Justine and Nicola as energetic and capable young women who packed an extraordinary amount into their lives.[392]

In Kate, the girls had a perfect role model. Their mother didn't have time for hobbies, but she loved cooking and entertaining. She was also a keen walker. For a few years in the early 1990s, though, she deviated from her preferred form of exercise to take up cycling. She may have done this to impress Neil, or simply to spend more time with him, for even though she was not a natural cyclist, she doggedly embraced the sport's particular challenges. Nicola and Justine were roped in too, and together the Jowell women cycled up and down the hills and vales of the city.

In 1990, and for three years thereafter, they participated in, and completed, Cape Town's famed cycle race, the Argus/Pick 'n Pay Cycle Tour. Then, in 1994, disaster struck, ending Kate's brief flirtation with cycling. While competing in her fourth 'Argus', she was involved in a pile-up, came off her bike and cracked her pelvis. The serious injury left her wheelchair-bound for two months, but she put on a brave face and continued to go about her business. This stoical approach prompted one of her admirers to add 'balls and guts' to the list of Kate's attributes.[393]

In retrospect, the accident was the start of a series of setbacks Kate faced in the mid-1990s. Unhappiness had settled on her life like a persistent fog. 'Things were not going the way she'd anticipated,' Justine says. It's possible she was also experiencing a mild form of 'empty nest syndrome': her daughters were growing up and were going their own ways. Justine matriculated in 1993 and Nicola in 1995, and they had both spent time travelling overseas. 'She was bitter. It was personal,' Justine says enigmatically. I sense that she is not willing to elaborate, and I don't press her. Professionally, Kate had also lost her edge, her sharpness. 'No one knew she was ill,' Justine elaborates, 'and while she must have known something was wrong, she was in denial for a long time.'[394]

For Justine, witnessing her mother's decline has been painful and harrowing. 'I try not to think about it,' she says, becoming tearful. Instead, she 'just gets on with things', often avoiding visiting Kate because it's simply too hard. 'I don't know if it's healthy … a part of me has already said goodbye to her, to the mother I knew, and I relate to her now as a different person,' she confesses, even though another part of her can't let go. Justine can't recall exactly when this change occurred. But, at the beginning of 2002, she went on a four-day retreat to Porterville to try to come to terms with the fact that her mother was dying.

As the crisis has deepened, Neil and his daughters have isolated, and insulated, themselves – from others, and also from one another. They have never really been a family that's talked openly about 'things like this,' Justine says. 'I think my dad would appreciate it on one level, but on another, I think he needs to be strong for us. So we help each other by not talking about it – which is probably not the best way to deal with my mother's illness.'[395]

Like Justine, Nicola – who, in 1996, had sent Kate a Mother's Day card thanking her for being 'the greatest and most understanding Mum!' – has battled to cope with her mother's decline. Living in the United Kingdom saved her for a time from watching Kate lose her grip on a meaningful existence. But the reprieve is temporary. Nicola has not escaped feelings of guilt and regret – for abandoning her mother at a time when Kate's life was closing in on her, and for leaving Justine and Neil to cope on their own. Nicola explains that she needed to make her own life choices: 'I hope, as we all do, that they are the right ones.'396

In fact, Kate's physician had urged the entire Jowell family to get on with their lives – even as Kate was being robbed of hers.

Nicola points out the painful paradox in her physical distance from Kate: it has cushioned her from witnessing Kate's deterioration on a daily or weekly basis, but when she does come home, it is all the more devastating to take in Kate's ever-worsening condition. 'Every time I have come home I have felt so unprepared for what I have encountered, and yet every time I hope that my mom will still know me, and we will be able to interact on some level.'

Acutely aware that she is fast losing touch with Kate, Nicola has found it hard to reconcile the person she now confronts with the mother she once knew. 'When I think of my future, and of Justine's – and what it might hold – I am now able to acknowledge that we will go through all our defining moments in life without my mom, and I realise that I miss her so very much. Alzheimer's does not give us permission to miss her – she is still with us. Yet we are grieving in a way that does not allow for closure.'397

During one of our very first conversations, Justine made the interesting revelation that Alzheimer's disease had 'softened' Kate's character in a 'beautiful' way. 'She's gentler and, in a lot of ways, easier now. In the past she was focused and driven, and now she's a lot mellower. The disease has also allowed her to connect differently with my dad, enabling him to be more loving, more supportive.'398

I ponder these things on my fifteen-minute trip from the Mouille Point café to the Jowells' home. Then, as I arrive at the house and pull into the driveway, my thoughts turn to Kate and I feel tense, wondering what kind of day she's having. Is she going to know who I am, and why I am visiting her? Is she going to be tired and confused? I press the doorbell. Eunice's muffled voice is just audible through the intercom. I push open the front door and head for the steep stairs that lead to the hub of the house.

During these past nine months, Kate has often met me at the bottom, excitement etched on her face, with some snippet of news to offer. But increasingly, it is the tall, wooden totem pole, a lonely, lean sculpture no doubt once chosen by Kate, that watches my guarded ascent.

I find Kate in her usual place, her eyrie, the informal open-plan lounge with its singular view of Table Bay and beyond. Her eyes are closed, and her head, heavy with sleep, drops forward, then jerks up as I greet her. She is momentarily startled before responding warmly to my arrival.

Eunice bustles in with her usual cheerful air. She's busy baking apricot muffins, she tells me, a weekly chore she's not particularly fond of because 'there are too many ingredients'. Bran rusks are her speciality, and also a broad, crusty health bread pockmarked with seeds. Both recipes come from Kate's once-considerable culinary repertoire.

Sitting on the couch, Kate seems small and shrunken. She is fading away; it's as if her mental withdrawal is matched by a physical one. Eunice reappears with a welcome tray of tea. She breaks Kate's rusk into uniform pieces. Placing one in Kate's hand, she tells her what it is. With a methodical single-mindedness, Kate eats all the pieces. Eunice pours her tea, then adds milk and sugar. 'Mrs Jowell, the tea is hot,' she warns, holding the cup to Kate's lips. Kate gulps thirstily. I notice then that her distinctive wedding ring, an unusually broad, angular yellow gold band, is no longer on her finger.

'Mrs Jowell doesn't wear it any more,' Eunice explains. 'She'd started pulling it off, and I'd often battle to find it. Now it just falls off because she's so thin.' Kate is oblivious to this development, to the fact that after thirty-three years, this piece of jewellery no longer signals her marital status. As Alzheimer's disease strips away her personality, so, too, material possessions are sloughed off.

Next to me, Kate repeatedly crosses and uncrosses her legs. Neil is overseas on business, and during his absence Eunice keeps watch over

Kate at night. For Kate's caregivers, the nights are the worst, as her sleep is disturbed. Like most sufferers of Alzheimer's disease, Kate wakes up several times at night and struggles to get back to sleep again. She also enjoys less and less deep sleep, the sleeping stage that is most restorative, and so she often feels tired. These changes in sleep patterns are thought to be due to neuron damage, and the loss of the brain's connecting pathways that bring about sleep.[399]

Increasingly, Kate naps during the day and restlessly wanders around at night.

In Justine's words, her 'ma' is 'disappearing'. 'It's becoming more and more difficult to connect with her. Her illness has become much more real, now,' she had told me just four months previously. For Nicola, whose only form of communication with her mother has till now been a long-distance telephone call, Kate's retreat into a silent world is a terrible absence – a kind of death.

~

While Kate's involvement in the labour world had waned considerably by the mid-1990s, in October of 1996 she was hand-picked by the Minister of Labour, Tito Mboweni, to serve on the Essential Services Committee along with respected Durban labour lawyer Dhaya Pillay and unionist Sunil Narian.

The chief concern of the committee, which operated under the auspices of the Commission for Conciliation, Mediation and Arbitration, was to determine whether certain services, including those rendered at hospitals, were essential or not.

In the feisty Dhaya Pillay, Kate found not only an intellectual equal – a strong woman used to speaking her mind – but an unlikely ally. Irrespective of their striking differences, or perhaps because of them, the pair struck up an immediate bond and their warm, vibrant friendship would continue long after they had completed the important task assigned to them.

'She made an impact on my life,' Dhaya confides. 'It was a very reassuring, comforting and confidence-building experience working with her.'[400]

Dhaya, the committee's chairperson, appreciated Kate's wealth of experience, even though she didn't have a legal background. Kate was fair-minded, objective and extremely professional, skills that perfectly complement Dhaya's own. On a personal level, Dhaya was impressed by Kate's honesty. 'I could rely on her instinct, her moral judgement and her criticism.'

The committee's brief, in part, was to conduct hearings on whether the dismantling of certain services would be life-threatening. The trio were charting a new course, and their committee was one of only three of its kind in the world.

During their tenure, they interacted with their counterparts in Italy and Canada, and the Italian connection particularly resonated with Kate. In fact, when I met her, one of the most vivid memories she had of her working life was a dramatic trip to Rome with Dhaya Pillay. Charming Italian men, glorious gastronomic excursions and a ride in a pert, olive Mini Cooper were uppermost in her mind.

Dhaya chuckles when I ask about the Cooper connection. 'It was a hilarious trip, which is why Kate can still remember it, especially the episode with that car!' The trip, in February 1998, was funded by the International Labour Organisation. Kate and Dhaya met with nine eminent Italian labour experts and sat in on their hearings. 'The chairman had a bell that he took great delight in ringing a great deal of the time. Kate's eyes popped out watching this strange way of doing business,' she recalls. After the hearings ended, Kate and Dhaya were duly invited to dine with the Italian committee. 'So there we were, following them out into this busy street where everyone triple-parks – and there, waiting in the gloaming, was this Mini Cooper, and it dawned on us that together with two very tall men we would have to fold ourselves into this tiny little car. It was a tight squeeze ... like something out of *Mr Bean*.'

In Italy, when they weren't studying the workings of the Italian labour system, the pair indulged in a shared passion for good food, and quickly made Garliano, a quaint little *ristorante* close to their hotel, their own. But, even though the trip – and the others the pair undertook – was profitable on a personal and professional level, it was clear to Dhaya that something was amiss in Kate's life.

'She was a pain in the neck when we travelled,' Dhaya says with characteristic candour, 'often losing things or forgetting about them completely.' Troubled, Dhaya put it down to Kate's busy lifestyle or that she was, perhaps, disorganised 'on that level' or simply getting old, until, finally, Kate confided in Dhaya that she was not well, that she was 'undergoing a series of tests'.

Kate's unravelling then became more and more obvious as she struggled to organise her life: faxes starting going astray, memos were lost.

In February 2000, Dhaya was appointed to the bench of the Labour Court and relinquished her committee duties. In any event, their work was done. 'Most of our work was concluded in three years. We basically worked ourselves out of a job!' Dhaya notes.

Then, they went their separate ways. Their firm friendship, however, would remain intact.

~

Kate Jowell's last year as director of the University of Cape Town's Business School in 1997 proved more than taxing. She was under relentless pressure, and it was obvious that she was taking strain.[401] She was often forgetful, and appeared tired. Her role as director had been denigrated by Mamphela Ramphele, the executive head of the university, who, it seems, did not believe Kate was up to the job. Says Norman Faull, 'After having worked incredibly hard, Kate was sent signals that she did not enjoy the support of the chief executive of the university.' The Business School's financial liability continued to be an issue, and Kate spent five years figuring out how to pay for the building, and how to cut the running costs of the Business School, instead of focusing on her other responsibilities as director.

She must certainly have felt despair, anger and frustration. But she never voiced her feelings. She was frequently subjected to what Norman Faull calls 'torrid sessions that were just horrible', where she would have to explain petty expenditures such as the Business School's electricity bill, and tea and coffee consumption, to the university's financial director. Yet Kate bore the full burden of financial accountability – even in its most trivial form. 'She was not a whinger,' Norman Faull points out.[402] To her great credit, Kate treated her persecutors with respect. 'She was a person of the highest integrity and fairness, and throughout this ordeal she was cordial and polite and proper,' Faull says.

As the months progressed, Faull saw his colleague getting progressively thinner, her face more drawn and taut each day. 'She really was in a no-win situation: unappreciated and unable to play to her strengths,' he recalls. Even though she did not voice it, Kate was taking enormous strain, and even though she must have tried to hide it, her life – and her health – had started to unravel. Clearly, she was run-down, exhausted, demoralised. And she must have been terribly lonely, too. Some of her colleagues and students put all this down to Kate's having too much on her plate. But those closest to her, including Mike Page and Yvonne van Stolk, were concerned that fatigue was not Kate's only health problem.

Page recalls a course in negotiation that Kate presented to the full-time 1997 MBA class, an exceptionally dynamic group of bright, keen go-getters. 'The students knew of her and were eager to experience her teaching first hand … but I know that they were disappointed, as she failed to live up to her reputation. By then, she was no longer the strong lecturer they had been expecting.'

While she continued to work with her students, an increasingly disconcerting change was occurring. For someone like Kate, the experience must have been especially unsettling and alarming. She confided in Van Stolk that often, during her lectures, she'd lose track of her argument. More and more, Kate became absent-minded, and mislaid things – in her office and elsewhere. Colleagues who approached her for important documents were often met with the perplexed response, 'It must be here somewhere.'

Yet her staff, ever loyal, covered for her. Van Stolk, realising that her once punctual boss could no longer keep track of time, bought an alarm clock for Kate and set it to ring five minutes before her appointments. Kate appreciated the gesture, and the alarm clock's intrusive shriek soon became a wry joke between the two women. Behind the laughter, however, Kate must surely have felt deeply troubled.

Still, Kate Jowell's illness was well hidden, John Simpson recalls.[403] Yet Simpson himself faced the fact a good three years before she resigned that something seemed to be very wrong with Kate Jowell. His once-alert colleague started to 'space out' at meetings. He was baffled. Kate had always been astute and focused. Her colleagues began to find it alarming attending meetings with her and listening to her wandering off the topic – if she grasped it at all. This was not the Kate Jowell they knew.

For Simpson, the turning point came when, in 1997, the Commerce Faculty asked the Business School to present a motivation to accompany a request for more funding. The strategic plan was presented by Mike Page, but it was all too obvious that he had not written it. Kate had written it, and it was a weak document. By now, the impact of her illness on her professional performance was dramatic. Clearly, Mike Page was covering for her, and faculty members were appalled and shocked, particularly by the implications of the presentation's poor content.

At the end of 1997, Kate threw in the towel and her tenure as director came to an abrupt end. She had accomplished an enormous amount, but her last months had been marred by her illness – which she herself still failed to acknowledge – and the enormous stress of her unhappy relationship with the powers-that-be at Bremner. Her last years as director – as a colleague noted in a farewell card signed 'Dave' – had been 'messy' and 'fairly thankless'. 'You deserve so much better,' he declared.

Her farewell function as Business School director – a modest tea in the staffroom – effectively ended a teaching career that had spanned more than two decades. The function was not attended by any of Kate's colleagues at Bremner, even though they had been invited. Mamphela Ramphele did not mark Kate's departure, nor did anyone from the

Commerce Faculty. This obvious slight angered many loyal friends and colleagues, who appreciated not only Kate's contributions, but also the sacrifices she had made.

'The function could have been far more special,' concedes Linda Fasham, the Business School's alumni relations manager. But the image of Kate battling to get through her speech remains with her. 'She stood there with a piece of paper in her hand, and she had to keep referring to it. This was not the Kate we had known, the woman who could address any gathering. It must have taken a lot of courage to do that. My heart went out to her.'[404]

Normal Faull concedes that no function, no matter how lavish or well attended, could have marked Kate's contribution, given the politics that beset the university and the Business School at the time. In his view, the University of Cape Town has repeatedly alienated some of its most faithful servants by undermining them.[405]

I imagine Kate clearing her office, taking down the artworks, retrieving her many books from the sagging melamine shelves. She may have stood on her balcony, watching students crossing the courtyard, remembering a time when a promising career lay before her. She must surely have felt bitter, disappointed, defeated.

Finally, I imagine her driving away from her alma mater in her old 7 Series metallic-gold BMW, leaving behind the squat white building with its glamorous view of her adopted city. Her heart must have been unbearably heavy.

~

The house is high up on a hill, at the end of a steep dirt road, and overlooks a picturesque range of mountains. The setting is New Hampshire, in the United States. For keen walkers like Kate Jowell, it's paradisal.

In December 1997, after vacating the director's chair, Kate received study and research leave from the University of Cape Town from January to December of the following year. During the sabbatical, she headed for the mountain retreat of her old friend Bob Rotberg and his wife, Joanna.

To the Rotbergs, Kate appeared for the most part to be 'very together'. However, she seemed very anxious about losing her way. Recalling the time, Rotberg says he should have realised then that Kate was displaying symptoms of Alzheimer's disease.

He explains: 'From the bottom of the driveway, you can take beautiful walks. If you turn left or right, you walk towards or away from a lovely lake, through the woods.' Kate would announce to the Rotbergs that she intended to take a walk. 'We'd say, "great",' and she'd say, "Which way do I go, left or right?" and a minute later she'd repeat the question.'[406]

When Kate returned to the university in 1999, it was clear that she was incapable of lecturing, even though she was keen to fulfil her duties. Mike Page felt the urge to protect her, from herself as much as from the vicious barbs of students and colleagues. 'It was clear that lecturing was too much to ask of her at that stage,' Page says.[407] He approached the Business School's new director, Professor Nick Segal, and suggested that Kate was no longer capable of carrying out her teaching duties. Segal agreed, and Kate, relieved of teaching responsibilities, dabbled in this and that. She must have felt lonely and terrified, having finally to acknowledge that, mentally and physically, she was on a steady decline. Where would it end?

Colleagues and friends were troubled by her condition. For Faull, there was a sense of horror that a relatively young, vibrant person had been struck down and somehow diminished in this way. 'It was really very difficult witnessing her becoming less of the person we had known for decades.'

In February 1998, at a staff meeting, it finally became clear to all her colleagues that Kate was not well. After an intense, prolonged discussion about a point on the agenda, Kate responded by telling the meeting that it was important for another point to be raised. Her request was met with shocked silence. 'The issue she raised was the very same one we had just spent about fifteen minutes heatedly debating,' Faull says.[408]

Page's concerns about Kate's health deepened, and the last straw came when he and Yvonne van Stolk accompanied her to lunch one day. Their former boss was keen to pick up the tab, but she battled to fill in the credit card slip and could not work out the tip for the waiter. Page and Van Stolk were shocked. This woman, a mathematician by training with a very quick business brain, was usually first to split the bill down to the last cent. Now she couldn't calculate a 10 per cent tip. Page took a chance and confided in her doctor, Jack Katz, about his concerns on the state of Kate's health.

Shortly afterwards, on 28 April 1999, Kate Jowell conceded that something had got the better of her, and took early retirement. Despite prevailing circumstances at the university, some colleagues did get to say goodbye to her, to wish her well, to thank her for her extraordinary contribution and the role she had played at the Business School. Many, like Norman Faull and Mike Page, realised that there was perhaps a certain logic to her departure. For after her tenure as director, returning to a life of lecturing would have been a backward move. Kate had realised her dream, she had made her mark. It was time for her to enjoy her life instead of pushing papers around at the Business School. But this realisation was overshadowed by a sense of sadness and tragedy at the ill-fated way her career – and her life – had come unstuck.

Kate herself retained her composure, not giving in to her emotions, even at this stage when she must surely have been smarting very badly. In a brief, moving letter to Nick Segal, she said, 'I write with some sadness to ask you to accept my wish to take early retirement from the Graduate School of Business with effect from the end of this month. As you are aware my health has not been good for some while and I have been advised by my doctor to retire.' The words, 'I will miss the GSB very much after twenty-five years' preceded her already somewhat shaky signature.

Soon afterwards, Neil and Kate told their daughters that she was terminally ill.

part six

AN UNCERTAIN WORLD

16

Home Alone

(1999–2009)

THEY HAD KNOWN that something was amiss, that Kate's world was out of kilter. But for Neil, Justine and Nicola, the naming of the affliction that had brought on Kate's painful humiliation and had led to her abandoning her career and extricating herself from society meant that they could no longer skirt around the issue.

On her birthday on 9 January, Justine and Nicola gave Kate a letter, penned on handmade paper, declaring that 1999 was going to be stress-free, 'a Kate year', where she would get a chance 'to take time out'. They would treat her to a sunset concert at Kirstenbosch Botanical Gardens, and yoga tuition for two months.

'We will accompany you some of the time ... we hope it gives you hours of wondrous relaxation, exercise and joy,' they wrote. But the stresses and strains remained. Kate didn't really take to yoga, mainly because she couldn't figure out what she had to do, Nicola says.[409] 'We all went for a while, then it petered out.'

Something was clearly amiss, and soon afterwards, during a mountain walk just behind Glencoe Road, Kate said as much to Justine. 'I had asked her how she was, and she became tearful and confessed that she had found out that she was ill,' Justine recalls.[410]

And it wasn't too long afterwards, with Neil at her side, that Kate revealed she had Alzheimer's. Justine no longer remembers her mother's exact words. 'We were sitting round the dinner table when she said she wanted to talk to us about something.' On hearing the news, Justine was worried and upset. Yet she was also relieved. 'At last there was an explanation for the fact that my mother had become someone I no longer knew,' Justine says.

Nicola reveals that Kate kept the news of her diagnosis to herself for a month, which must have been excruciating. 'She was diagnosed in May 1999, and she told us a month later,' Nicola says.[411] 'She broke down and cried. We all cried.' By that time Nicola had matriculated from St Cyprian's and had spent a year at the Cordon Bleu Cookery School in England. She was completing a Social Science undergraduate degree at UCT. Later she would follow her heart and return to the United Kingdom in 2002.

Kate had retreated to Glencoe Road, yet she still had fight in her. She tried to forge a new existence, to reassert herself in her world, counting on her interests to help her pass the time and prop up her crumbling life. She gardened, brushed up on her French, joined eminent Cape Town cosmologist (and avid walker) George Ellis on mountain hikes, spent time with her mother and her daughters. In the most obvious material manifestation of this need, she sold her trusty old BMW and replaced it with a sleek, berry-coloured Audi.

But Alzheimer's closed in on her. Kate had not enjoyed driving the new car for long before it became obvious that she was a danger on the road. Unable to judge distances, she often became confused and nervous. Her family shied away from robbing her of her autonomy; nonetheless, as Nicola notes, being in the car when she was driving was terrifying.[412] Eunice confirms this, saying that she became aware of just how much Kate's driving had deteriorated when, on a trip to the station, 'the car behind us hooted at us all the time'.[413] Finally, Kate's neurologist, John Gardiner, stepped in and gave her an ultimatum: if she had an accident, he would be obliged to tell the authorities that he had long since advised her to stop driving.

And so Kate's isolation deepened, as did her vulnerability. On one occasion, on an outing with her driver, she stopped at a delicatessen and came away with a piece of imported cheese that cost her R250. Later, when Neil discovered the purchase, he 'had a heart attack', as Nicola puts it. 'It's of great concern that people can take advantage of her in this way,' Nicola says, recalling the incident.[414]

On 10 August 2000, Kate received an email from Bob Rotberg and his wife, Joanna, asking after her health and enquiring if she was up to meeting a New York friend of theirs who was due to travel to Cape Town. 'How are you about social things?' Rotberg wrote. 'Shall I urge her to find you or will it be too taxing?'

Kate replied, through Neil's PA Patricia Love, that 'somehow' she was managing to function normally, attend a few board meetings, and that she and Neil would be 'delighted' to entertain the Rotbergs' friend in Cape Town. Yet, in spite of Kate's assurances, the email is filled with clues that all is not well: the wording is clumsy, and several blank spaces on the typed version show that Love battled to decipher Kate's deteriorating handwriting.

After offering the news that her mother had recently suffered a small stroke, Kate urged Joanna – who herself had not been well – never to give up. 'Don't ever give up is right,' Rotberg replied. 'We are so glad you are functioning well.'

The Rotbergs' friend, Professor Susan Woodward, was an expert on the Balkans, and this would be her first visit to Africa. Delighted that the Jowells would 'give her some hospitality', Rotberg said, 'I am sure that you will like her … she is only a little younger than you.' In pencil, Kate added a cheeky rejoinder: 'Therefore too old to be of interest to NIJ.' Clearly, her sense of humour was still intact.

But yet another blow awaited Kate. In 2002, Kathleen Bowman died. For some years she'd been living in Cape Town, in a complex in Mouille Point, overlooking the sea. Kate was devastated by her mother's death, Paul says, and at her memorial, when a small crowd gathered to pay their last respects, at Kathleen's request a rendition of the song 'Goodbye Kathleen' rang out in the cold Cape Town air. Shortly afterwards, Kate resigned from all her remaining professional commitments – most notably from the board of directors of insurance giant Sanlam. At a special farewell she was presented with a 1620s Blaeu map of Africa.

~

December 2003. 'It's as if she's gone, even though, physically, she's still here.' Eunice becomes tearful; the house, she says, 'is so empty without her'. The Mrs Jowell she'd known and confided in is no longer there. The woman who took an interest in her life and her family is gone, leaving behind what writer Sue Miller calls 'a needier and needier husk, a kind of animated shell requiring attention and care'.[415] Eunice, resolute and loyal, suddenly declares: 'I will never leave Mrs Jowell now, because she's been very good to me.'

For Paul Bowman, who has not seen his sister for a few months, her decline is even more alarming. 'She is not in touch with anything any more. She can't stand properly or eat on her own.'[416] For me, though, the most startling sign that Kate has turned a corner is the sudden disappearance of her handbag. In itself an anomaly, the rectangular black satin evening clutch bag Kate had always reached for just before our routine departures for Carlucci's symbolised a life sadly out of sync. Its inappropriateness, the fact that it held nothing more than a credit card, that it was kept in a kitchen cupboard – these were poignant indications that the conventions of ordinary life had ceased to matter to her because, increasingly, they had ceased to register.

There's a certain dull obviousness to the disappearance of the bag: Kate can no longer hold a pen, let alone commit so much as a squiggle to a credit card slip. Yet I feel its absence acutely.

Now that it's gone, the bag can only stand for the loss of our friendship, which was fading even as it began.

Kate's other friendships, like her memory, have all but been obliterated. Most of Kate's crew have jumped ship a long time ago. Even the committed Capricorns, Gorry Bowes Taylor and Annette Kesler, don't come round or call any more.

Judge Dhaya Pillay, who is based in Durban, phones Neil from time to time, as does Yvonne Galombik. Mike Page, Trevor Williams and Robert Rotberg connect with Kate through my sporadic emails. It is hardly surprising. It takes courage to keep up with a friend whose existence is being shredded by a disease like Alzheimer's.

～

January 2006. A surprising email from one of Kate's former students, Ken McKenzie, who also worked at UCT administration and was 'a sometime guest lecturer' at the Business School, lands in my inbox. 'I want to make contact with Kate, to say "hi" and connect on a human level,' he says. 'I know she has been struck down by Alzheimer's. I suspect that old friends and colleagues drop you when this happens.'[417] He wonders if his meeting Kate would cause her distress or embarrassment. I explain that Kate will not be able to communicate with him in a meaningful way, as her illness is far advanced. He backs off, and says that under the circumstances 'it is probably best for me to leave Kate in peace – although one never knows for sure'. I immediately regret his decision. Kate might well enjoy his visit. Neil agrees, and we start to sort out suitable times and dates.

Sadly, due to bad timing, the visit doesn't happen. But I ask Ken for his recollections of his former lecturer. 'I remember Kate as beautiful, sharp-witted and occasionally sharp-tongued with any dumb, sexist MBA student. I think we were all partly in love with her – and partly terrified of her, too.'[418]

A few months later, I have a similar conversation with Naas Steenkamp, Kate's friend and former fellow National Manpower Commission member. Soon he is making his way from his home in Somerset West to Glencoe Road, armed with flowers and a 'neat little card' bearing the words, 'To my very dear Kate, from your friend Naas, *amicus semper.*'

On his way, he ponders their chequered history. How much time has slipped by without contact. He wonders if Kate is going to know who he is and why I had told him Neil would be delighted by his visit. Why not Kate? 'Is Kate resentful that I am one of those who simply faded away? Worse, does she perhaps not remember me?'

I do not warn Naas that, in fact, his journey to see Kate will be more about saying goodbye than renewing a friendship. At this late stage of Alzheimer's, Kate has no system of retrieving her and Naas's shared memories.

Indeed. The Kate he encounters on arriving at Glencoe Road is a shadow of her former self. The silent woman who shuffles next to Neil 'head down, face averted' is not the Kate he knew. She is not the dark-haired beauty in the flimsy yellow dress who created a stir in the auditorium of the Laboria Building in Pretoria.

Later, making sense of his visit in a beautiful, cathartic piece of writing, Naas confesses to watching Kate's compulsive ritual of crossing and uncrossing her legs after Neil helps her into her chair. At a loss for words, he is unsure of how to reach her.

> *'Those* omies *of the commission used to call you the rose among the thorns, Kate,' I start, not knowing where I am heading, but determined to go on. I'm unsure of my emotions. Anguish such as I have long not felt, yes, but despair, a rising sense of hysteria, an urge to flee. But here sits the solid, fragile Neil, now my buttress. I also feel a resolve. I'm going to get through to Kate, kindle a recognition of something, warm her heart, even if the moment flickers only briefly. Because I have been noticing something in these last strained minutes. Kate seems to be listening. Listening intently, with utterly focused concentration. Concentration! She was always so good at it. I talk.*

Naas tells her that she was a prophet of reconciliation, that he learnt a huge amount from her; he draws on their well of memories, reminding her of mundane things, of great initiatives, of the colourful people they encountered at econo-political risk analyst Anna Starcke's salon. His efforts are rewarded when, unexpectedly, Kate slowly lifts her head and looks at him with eyes that are dark, unfathomable. 'They are not quizzical, yet I sense them probing me. She looks at me for what feels like a long minute before averting her face.'

Encouraged, Naas cheerily recounts the day when she 'set the crowd abuzz', telling her that she entered the auditorium against the sun, wearing her yellow dress that was 'actually rather transparent'. He stops talking, detecting a slight stirring in Kate, a minute movement. 'Then, from somewhere within, comes a word, unmodulated, husky, but clear. "Yes," says Kate. A moment passes in which we are immobile, Kate, Neil and I. I look up at Neil. He has tears in his eyes.'

~

January 2007. We are a motley crew, gathered at Glencoe Road for a tea to mark Kate's sixty-seventh birthday: Neil, Justine and Nicola, Lindy Smit, me, Yvonne van Stolk, Patricia Swanepoel – Neil's PA, formerly Patricia Love – and Eunice. Alzheimer's is the unwanted, uninvited guest. Painfully thin, hunched and withdrawn, Kate still clings tenaciously to what we can only assume is a dreadful life.

I watch her as she crosses and uncrosses her thin legs, and then suddenly leans over to bite her knee. Eunice hovers. Occasionally Kate makes eye contact, answering a question with a slight smile or a monosyllabic 'yes' or 'no'. But mostly she is mute as the chatter swirls around her. Her grey hair, cropped short, caps her bony skull. Restlessly, her right hand finds her tongue.

She is oblivious to the fact that Nicola returned from the United Kingdom to live in Cape Town two years ago; that she has bought a house in Vredehoek, close to Justine, and has recently got engaged to her partner, Philip Brink. Kate is unaware, too, that she has missed not only the plotting and planning of Justine's wedding to Ross Frylinck – whom she had a chance to meet before Alzheimer's tightened its grip – but the joyous occasion itself, which took place on 23 April 2005 at the family's farm on the Wedderwill Estate near Somerset West.

By the time the rainy day dawned, Justine was 'kind of prepared' for the fact that her mother would not witness her unconventional wedding to Ross. As she puts it, Kate had slowly been stepping out of her life, being progressively unable to share her thoughts and dilemmas, or engage with her on an emotional, spiritual or intellectual level.

'Ross and I spent a lot of time reflecting on our wedding and our marriage long before it happened. I had a chance to think a lot about marriage in general, my parents' relationship, my relationship with my mom and her deteriorating illness – and what Ross and I wanted to create for ourselves in our own lives.'[419]

For Justine, the experience was emotionally hard, yet grounding. 'I am incredibly grateful for having had the chance to come to terms with these things … it really helped to prepare me for the enormity of the next step Ross and I were taking, the role my mom could no longer play in my life and how hard it might be in the future.'

But by far the hardest part was wondering how much Kate was able to understand and whether she felt excluded and left out, 'waiting at home while we were out celebrating an event she would have loved to attend'. Justine still wonders about it, and about other similar times when Kate has been excluded from family celebrations.

Paul's presence at the wedding was comforting for Justine, though, and she consciously wore one of her favourite pieces of Kate's jewellery, a striking necklace of old amber beads. 'I think, if it's possible, that she was there in spirit, and I know that she would have acknowledged and hopefully appreciated our wedding and the vows we made to each other.'

~

January 2009. Kate's birthday tea is in full swing. We are all there, like old faithfuls, to wish her well and share her favourite chocolate cake: Neil, Justine and Nicola, Lindy Smit, Yvonne van Stolk, Patricia Swanepoel and Eunice. Paul Bowman, Kate's brother, is a welcome addition to the party.

Kate is looking fragile but well. While she can no longer walk, she still gets dressed every day and wiles away the hours in the open-plan informal lounge. She is no longer able to focus on the dramatic cityscape view or the wide expanse of blue sea just beyond, and it is hard to know what respite the long days offer. She has lost the use of her left hand and arm after suffering, presumably, a light stroke or series of strokes a while ago. So it is her right hand that compulsively tugs at the hem of her pants, pulling it above her bony knee and back down again.

The week before Paul's arrival, Lindy had reminded Kate, who now requires twenty-four-hour care, that her brother was on his way from Florida. 'I got a response,' Lindy says, smiling. She is convinced that Kate still has lucid moments, even if they're few and far between, revealed through the flicker of an eye, a slight smile or the odd spoken word. In this way, Lindy resolutely keeps Kate in touch with her world and her family. 'She's still there ... she's still a part of their lives,' she says. 'I have told her that the girls are married now and that she's about to become a grandma!'[420]

A comforting presence in Kate's life since 2002, Lindy, in fact, suggested to Kate she needed to tell her life story. 'I thought it would be therapeutic, and at the time she had things she wanted other people to know about Alzheimer's.' For Kate, it was a case of living with Alzheimer's, not dying from it. 'She felt there was something she could still do, and working on a book gave her a sense of purpose.'

Lindy, a social worker in private practice who sits on the board of Dementia SA and Action on Elder Abuse SA, has managed Kate's Alzheimer's every step of the way, becoming a crucial link between the patient 'who crept into my heart', her family and her caregivers.

It has not been an easy road to travel, though. Initially Kate found Lindy's visits difficult because they reminded her of her illness. 'She was open about having Alzheimer's, but reserved, and I had to move beyond the reserve to reach her, to get glimpses of the real Kate,' Lindy says. 'It's also been very difficult watching her physical deterioration, knowing there is nothing you can do to stop it other than be there for her and try to make her as comfortable as possible.'

At the heart of Lindy's caring philosophy is the premise that Kate's caregivers 'remember who she is' and put her needs first. The focus, always, is on Kate, not on Alzheimer's disease. She has taught Eunice – and the carers who relieve her when she takes a well-deserved break – to anticipate Kate's needs because she cannot express them herself.

Lindy has also kept a watchful eye on Kate's caregivers so that they don't succumb to burnout, exhaustion, depression, stress and loneliness. 'As a caregiver you can't expect rewards and recognition for your efforts – you have to be selfless,' Lindy muses. You also can't expect any feedback. But there are times when you do get a flicker of recognition. 'It keeps me going ... and it keeps Eunice going too.'

For Lindy, her time with Kate has been rewarding. She feels privileged to have known her, to have walked down this rocky, debilitating road with her. 'Throughout her ordeal she's remained a lady, and I have learnt a lot from her about just how much the human body can endure.'[421]

~

July 2009. 'I feel I should be saying or doing the things Kate would have said or done,' Neil says, looking slightly forlorn.[422] He has just returned from a week-long trip to France to see his sons Paul and David – and has just missed the very premature birth of Joseph, Justine and Ross's firstborn.

Kate, too, has missed this dramatic arrival of her first grandchild. She has been robbed of watching her daughter become a mother, of being part of celebrating another joyous family milestone. Last year she also missed the marriage of her youngest daughter.

For a while I have been nudging Nicola to think about her wedding day and the impact of Kate's absence from her life. I have almost given up when this touching email arrives one wintry Cape Town morning.

Philip Brink and I got married on 26 April 2008 after knowing each other for about eight years. Not having my mom around during the initial stages of our relationship was a strange experience. She met Philip for the first time at a birthday dinner in January 2001. By this time she was already seriously ill and was not the Kate she'd still been a couple of years before.

Philip had heard a lot about her from people he knew, and I think he must have had certain expectations. It will always be a source of great sadness that they were not given an opportunity to get to know one another. I think – rather, I know – they would have got on well. My mom would have enjoyed Philip's sharp wit and passionate nature. Once, on leaving the house after a visit a couple of months ago, Eunice turned to me and said, 'She would have approved of the two of you.' As usual, I felt tears welling up. I realised I have not really thought about how different things would have been had she not succumbed to Alzheimer's.

I went about planning our wedding in my usual head-down manner of getting things done, making lists and notes, of which I am sure my mom would have been very proud! I usually push things I don't want to deal with to the back of my mind. That Ma would not be around during the run-up to the wedding, or on the day, was something I edged firmly behind all the other pressing issues on my mind – it was well hidden away!

Nonetheless I often felt sad that she wasn't there to talk things through with me, to give me the reassurance that I needed, or perhaps spoil the bride-to-be. It was in the weeks before the wedding, while talking with our marriage officer, that the full emotional effect of it all came tumbling out.

The week before the big day we decided that Justine would light a special candle at the start of the ceremony in memory of Ma. This turned into a very poignant moment during the ceremony, and was a very important way of acknowledging the person who was present by her very absence.

When Justine got married, there was some discussion about Ma coming to her wedding. At that point, she was not well enough to attend, and had already been home-bound for a long time. But iron-ically, it was this sense that we needed to keep trying to include her in our lives that eventually led us to decide she should not attend – a decision we all knew was the right one. In some way it was a relief to me on the day of my wedding that, although we all wanted her to be there, we were spared making that hard decision.

My dad has often spoken of the conversations he had with my mother when she got sick. He was always tearful when recounting her sadness and her biggest fear – that she would not get to see us marry and have children, and establish our careers. She would not see us as the adults we would eventually become. And when I think of my life now and my wedding day, I realise that she left us so early – I can't quite remember the last milestone in my life of which she would have been aware.

I think she would have loved our wedding. It was a beautiful April day and it took place at Wedderwill, our family farm outside Somerset West. Although the morning started out cold and cloudy, it blossomed into the most beautiful of days. I realise Ma no longer knew the person who was getting married or half the people there or, sadly, even the location. Wedderwill came into the family around the time she was diagnosed, and she did not really spend much time there.

However, I know she would have loved the fact that we did it our way, with people who were important to us. We designed a casual ceremony that was set in the middle of the veld overlooking the valley below. The content was valuable to us as we had written each other's vows. I remember arriving at the ceremony quite a way away, and I had a long walk to the point where I met up with my dad, who would walk me down the aisle, and to Justine.

When I reached them, I realised that Neil was very emotional, and how difficult this moment was for him. Was it because, after attending the weddings of his four other children, this was the first time he was escorting a bride down the aisle? Was it nerves? Or was it the beauty of the surroundings and the emotion he felt for me? But of course he was once again witnessing one of the special moments in his family's life without Ma, and his sadness had as much to do with him as it did with her.

I don't know what I expected on that long walk towards Philip – words of encouragement or praise, perhaps some last-minute advice on the next phase of my life. Instead I found myself trying to comfort Pa as he struggled to control his emotions.

The ceremony was beautiful, and the lighting of the candle in Ma's honour was a perfect tribute. I managed to keep my emotions in check until the vows, when the tears started to come – due to excitement and nerves, but also the realisation of the gap in my life.

I think Ma would have been very proud of the person I have become, even though there are areas where we would have stumbled or clashed as only a mother and daughter can. She became ill before I really became an adult and started on my own journey in life. So it is difficult to know how we would have related to each other now or the role that she would have played in my life. I was always the child who needed a lift somewhere or some spending money!

Philip and I now own our own business, and I know that she would have loved that – we spoke about it while I was at school, as she recognised that it was tough in South Africa and creating your own future was so important. I think I spent a long time wanting to follow in her footsteps and feeling that there was an expectation for me to do so – not necessarily from immediate family. So I think she would have been very encouraging about the steps I am taking now. But one thing I know for sure: I wouldn't mind her advice right now!

For Nicola and Justine, Kate's Alzheimer's has probably exacerbated what Sue Miller identifies as 'a lifelong feeling of loss'. While Miller concedes that it was Alzheimer's that finally took her own father away, he had, in fact, 'long since been taken': he'd been gone, claimed elsewhere by his beliefs and convictions years before, when she was growing up. [423] In a similar sense, Kate had also 'long since [been] taken' from her daughters – claimed by her ambitions, her career, her success.

And so it is as if the Jowell daughters are paying a double price: having lost their mother once, they have had to watch her moving inexorably away once again – though this time, 'step by step into a dementing illness'. As Miller poignantly says, 'it's hard not to want to blame someone – ourselves most of all'.

Epilogue

I T WAS NEVER my intention to present Kate Jowell as 'the Alzheimer's lady', which, as British biographer AN Wilson points out, has become the fate of the late Iris Murdoch. In his biography of the well-known British writer and philosopher, he talks of 'the dark that would engulf her last days' and of 'the distortion of her image in the public mind by various books, and by the film'. She was doomed, he says, to become 'the Alzheimer's lady', and her memory is now perpetuated not only by her extraordinary contribution to English, but also by the disease that killed her.

But it was perhaps inevitable that the disease – which has exerted so potent an influence on the Jowells' family life – would come to define Kate.

She is an enigma to the end: in a rare moment when she looks up, her eyes are piercing, but most times they are vacant. Who knows what she is thinking or feeling, and if she is able to think or feel at all. Though I have watched Kate closely over the years, I have not managed to prise out her secret. Yet I am so much the richer for the experience, and as AN Wilson said of a similar misgiving he had about Iris Murdoch, in the end 'it really does not matter'.[424]

Sharon Sorour-Morris
August 2009

Notes

PROLOGUE

1. Kate Jowell, interview, Cape Town, 31.1.2003.
2. Neil Jowell, interview, Cape Town, 2.4.2003.
3. As quoted in Zelda Gordon-Fish, 'The Director's Chair', *Cosmopolitan*, October 1993, p. 54.
4. As quoted in Gorry Bowes Taylor, 'Bird Brain', *Woman's Argus*, 28 February 1974.
5. Interviews with confidential sources.
6. William Molloy and Paul Caldwell, *Alzheimer's Disease* (London: Robinson, 2002), p. 17.
7. Mick Jackson, *The Underground Man* (London: Picador, 1998), p. 33.
8. John Bayley, *Iris: A Memoir of Iris Murdoch* (Great Britain: Abacus, 1999), p. 277.

CHAPTER 1

9. Paul Bowman, telephone interview, 3.3.2003.
10. Leslie Stone, telephone interview, Knysna, 7.7.2003.

11. Paul Bowman, telephone interview, 3.2.2003, *op. cit.*
12. Kate Jowell, interview, Cape Town, 12.3.2003.
13. Leslie Stone, telephone interview, Knysna, 7.7.2003.

CHAPTER 2

14. Alexandra Fuller, *Don't Let's Go to the Dogs Tonight* (London: Picador, 2002), p. 39.
15. Paul Bowman, interview, Cape Town, 3.3.2003.
16. *Ibid.*
17. Neil Jowell, interview, Cape Town, 12.3.2003.
18. Kate Jowell, interview, Cape Town, 5.3.2003.
19. Leslie Stone, telephone interview, Knysna, 7.7.2003.
20. Kate Jowell, interview, Cape Town, 5.3.2003.
21. DC Browning, *Everyman's English Dictionary* (London: J.M. Dent & Sons, no date).
22. Paul Bowman, interview, Cape Town, 3.3.2003.

CHAPTER 3

23. Kate Jowell, interview, Cape Town, 30.5.2003.
24. Kate Jowell, interview, Cape Town, 8.1.2003.
25. Gorry Bowes Taylor, interview, Cape Town, 24.1.2003.
26. As quoted in Zelda Gordon-Fish, *op. cit.*, p. 56.
27. As quoted in Gorry Bowes Taylor, *op. cit.*
28. Zelda Gordon-Fish, *op. cit.*, p. 56.
29. Kate Jowell, interview, Cape Town, 17.2.2003.
30. Doris Hollander, telephone interview, London, 19.5.2003.
31. Zelda Gordon-Fish, *op. cit.*, p. 56.
32. *Ibid.*

CHAPTER 4

33. *TIME* magazine, quoted in *Junior Chronicle of the 20th Century* (London: Dorling Kindersley, 1997), p. 204.
34. Paul Bowman, email interview, 19.7.2003.
35. Salisbury was the capital of Rhodesia at the time. Its name changed to Harare after independence in 1980.
36. Paul Bowman, telephone interview, Florida, United States, 3.3.2003.
37. *Junior Chronicle of the 20th Century*, p. 204.
38. *Ibid.*
39. Neil Jowell, interview, Cape Town, 12.3.2003.
40. Paul Bowman, interview, Cape Town, 12.5.2003.
41. Neil Jowell, interview, Cape Town, 12.3.2003.

42. Kate Jowell, interview, Cape Town, 6.1.2003.
43. William Molloy and Paul Caldwell, *op. cit.*, p. 29.
44. Nicola Jowell, interview, Cape Town, 11.1.2003.
45. Justine Jowell, interview, Cape Town, 21.2.2003.
46. Justine Jowell, interview, Cape Town, 5.3.2003.
47. William Molloy and Paul Caldwell, *op. cit.*, p. 31.
48. *Ibid.*
49. Kate Jowell, interview, Cape Town, 31.1.2003.
50. William Molloy and Paul Caldwell, *op. cit.*, p. 17.
51. Sue Miller, *The Story of My Father* (New York: Alfred A. Knopf, 2003), p. 69.
52. William Molloy and Paul Caldwell, *op. cit.*, p. 7.
53. *Ibid.*
54. Paul Bowman, interview, Cape Town, 12.5.2003.
55. *Ibid.*

CHAPTER 5

56. As quoted in Jane Raphaely, 'Last word', *Fairlady*, 5 July 2000, p. 88.
57. *Ibid.*
58. Associated Magazines, with its headquarters in Cape Town, publishes *Cosmopolitan, House and Leisure, O – The Oprah Magazine* and *Marie Claire.*
59. *South Africa in the 20th Century* (Cape Town: Struik, 2000), p. 149.
60. Sue MacGregor, *Woman of Today*, (London: Headline, 2002), p. 93.

61. *Ibid.*

62. Sue MacGregor, email interview, 21.8.2003.

63. Sue MacGregor was made an Officer of the Order of the British Empire (OBE) in 1992, and a Commander of the Order of the British Empire (CBE) in 2002.

64. Sue MacGregor, email interview, 21.8.2003.

65. Jenny le Roux, interview, Cape Town, 24.5.2003.

66. Sally Graaff, telephone interview, Cape Town, 15.6.2003.

67. Sue MacGregor, email interview, 22.8.2003.

68. Albie Sachs, interview, Clifton, Cape Town, 30.8.2003.

69. Kate Jowell, interview, Cape Town, 3.9.2003.

70. Albie Sachs, interview, 30.8.2003.

71. Jane Raphaely, *op. cit.*

72. Cathy Knox, telephone interview, Grahamstown, 13.8.2003.

73. *Ibid.*

74. *Fair Lady*, March, 1965.

75. Jenny le Roux, interview, Cape Town, 24.5.2003.

76. Jane Raphaely, interview, Cape Town, 2.2.2003.

77. As quoted in Eileen Snowball, 'Memories are made of this ...' *Fairlady*, 5 July 2000, p. 21.

78. Jane Raphaely, interview, Cape Town, 23.7.2003.

79. Eileen Snowball, *op. cit.*

80. Cathy Knox, telephone interview, Grahamstown, 13.8.2003.

81. From www.bibacollection.com.

82. Kate Jowell, interview, Cape Town, 17.2.2003.

83. Albie Sachs, interview, Cape Town, 30.8.2003.

84. Cathy Knox, telephone interview, Grahamstown, 13.8.2003.

CHAPTER 6

85. Neil Jowell, interview, Cape Town, 26.5.2003.

86. Albie Sachs, interview, Cape Town, 30.8.2003.

87. One such occasion was an interview I had with her in Cape Town on 30.5.2003.

88. Jane Raphaely, interview, Cape Town, 2.2.2003.

89. Neil Jowell, interview, Cape Town, 26.5.2003.

90. Albie Sachs, interview, 30.8.2003.

91. Confidential source, interview, Cape Town, 15.6.2003.

92. Jenny le Roux, interview, Cape Town, 24.5.2003.

93. Kate Jowell, interview, Cape Town, 17.3.2003.

94. Phyllis Jowell, assisted by Adrienne Folb, *Joe Jowell of Namaqualand – The Story of a Modern-day Pioneer* (Cape Town: Fernwood Press, 1994).

95. *Ibid.*

96. Neil Jowell, interview, Cape Town, 8.9.2003.

97. Anneliese Kuhn, 'Men with Millions', *Scope*, 5 March 1971, p. 90.

98. *Ibid.*

99. *Ibid*, p. 91.

100. As quoted in Phyllis Jowell, *op. cit.*

101. As quoted in Phyllis Jowell, *op. cit.*, p. 263.

102. As quoted in Anneliese Kuhn, *op. cit.*, p. 90.

103. Neil Jowell, interview, Cape Town, 26.5.2003.

104. Kate Jowell, interview, Cape Town, 30.5.2003.

105. Paul Bowman, email interview, 12.6.2003.

CHAPTER 7

106. Foreword to David Shenk, *The Forgetting – Understanding Alzheimer's: A Biography of a Disease* (London: HarperCollins, 2001), p. ix.

107. *Ibid.*

108. William Molloy and Paul Caldwell, *op. cit.*, p. 61.

109. *Ibid.*

110. Jane Raphaely, interview, Cape Town, 2.2.2003.

111. David Shenk, *op. cit.*, p. 32.

112. Lin Sampson, telephone interview, Cape Town, 11.11.2003.

113. Sydney Baker, telephone interview, Greece, 22.8.2003.

114. Annette Kesler, interview, Cape Town, 7.7.2003.

115. Jane Raphaely, email interview, Cape Town, 1.6.2009.

116. Neil Jowell, interview, Cape Town, 26.5.2003.

117. As quoted in Gorry Bowes Taylor, *op. cit.*

118. Sydney Baker, telephone interview, Greece, 22.8.2003.

119. Confidential source, telephone interview, Cape Town, 12.11.2003.

120. Paul Bowman, interview, Cape Town, 29.10.2003.

121. Jenny le Roux, interview, Cape Town, 24.5.2003.

122. Jane Raphaely, interview, Cape Town, 2.2.2003.

123. In David Shenk, *op. cit.*, p. xii.

CHAPTER 8

124. As quoted in Zelda Gordon-Fish, *op. cit.*, p. 56.

125. As quoted in Gorry Bowes Taylor, *op. cit.*, p. 2.

126. *Ibid.*

127. Phyllis Jowell, *op. cit.*, p. 246.

128. Neil Jowell, interview, Cape Town, 26.5.2003.

129. Gorry Bowes Taylor, *op. cit.*, p. 2.

130. Meyer Feldberg, telephone interview, New York City, 14.1.2004.

131. As quoted in *The Cape Times Homefinder*, Saturday, 24 September 1977.

132. Phyllis Jowell, *op. cit.*, p. 280.

133. *Ibid.*, p. 281.

134. Harris Gordon, telephone interview, Cape Town, 5.6.2003.

135. Kate Jowell, interview, Cape Town, 12.3.2003.

136. David Shenk, *op. cit.*, p. 115.

137. *Ibid.*

138. *Ibid.*, p. 118.

139. *Ibid.*

140. *Ibid.*

141. Gorry Bowes Taylor, *op. cit.*, p. 2.

142. *Ibid.*

143. Neil Jowell, interview, Cape Town, 12.3.2003.

144. John Simpson, interview, Cape Town, 12.3.2003.

CHAPTER 9

145. Zelda Gordon-Fish, *op. cit.*, p. 58.
146. Michael Morris, *Every Step of the Way* (Cape Town: Human Sciences Research Council, 2004), p. 212.
147. *Ibid.*, p. 213.
148. *Ibid.*
149. Kate Jowell, 'Labour Policy in South Africa', *The South African Journal of Economics*, 47.4, 1979, p. 375.
150. Michael Morris, *op. cit.*, p. 213.
151. *Ibid.*, p. 371.
152. As quoted in Godfrey de Bruyn, 'Kate Jowell: Informed and Perceptive', *Sun*, January 1987, p. 12.
153. *Ibid.*
154. Zelda Gordon-Fish, *op. cit.*, p. 58.
155. Kate Jowell, as quoted in Gorry Bowes Taylor, 'Managing It', *The Argus*, 13 March 1979.
156. *Finance Week*, 3–9 May 1979, p. 531.
157. *Ibid.*
158. John Simpson, interview, Cape Town, 18.12.2003.
159. Gorry Bowes Taylor, 'Managing It', *op. cit.*
160. Neil Jowell, interview, Cape Town, 12.5.2009.
161. Kate Jowell, 'Labour Policy in South Africa', *op. cit.*, p. 376.
162. Zelda Gordon-Fish, op. cit., p. 58.
163. Kate Jowell, 'Labour Policy in South Africa', *op. cit.*, p. 390.
164. *Ibid.*
165. *Ibid.*
166. *Ibid.*, p. 393.
167. *Ibid.*
168. *Ibid.*, p. 394.
169. *Ibid.*
170. *Ibid.*, p. 395.
171. *Ibid.*
172. *Ibid.*, p. 396.
173. Kate Jowell, as quoted in 'Management "must learn to negotiate"', *Cape Times*, 1 December 1979.
174. *Ibid.*
175. SP Botha, 'Inquiry Members', *Cape Times*, 1 November 1979.
176. 'Manpower Commission – Women Vastly Outnumbered,' *The Star*, 2 November 1979.
177. *Ibid.*
178. *Ibid.*
179. *Ibid.*
180. As quoted in Gorry Bowes Taylor, 'Women in Labour', *op. cit.*
181. *Ibid.*
182. Kate Jowell, as quoted in 'Bias exists against women – lecturer', *The Argus*, 8 October 1979.
183. *Ibid.*
184. *Ibid.*
185. Neil Jowell, interview, 26.5.2004.
186. *Ibid.*
187. *Ibid.*
188. Kate Jowell, as quoted in Gorry Bowes Taylor, 'Managing It', *op. cit.*
189. Nicola Jowell, interview, Cape Town, 11.1.2003.
190. Justine Jowell, interview, Cape Town, 21.2.2003.
191. Nicola Jowell, interview, 11.1.2003.
192. Neil Jowell, interview, Cape Town, 12.3.2003.
193. Jannie Graaff, interview, Cape Town, 10.2.2004.
194. Neil Jowell, interview, 12.3.2003.
195. Kate Jowell, as quoted in Gorry Bowes Taylor, 'Managing It', *op. cit.*

196. Yvonne Galombik, interview, Cape Town, 13.2.2004.
197. Kate Jowell, as quoted in Gorry Bowes Taylor, 'Managing It', *op. cit.*
198. William Molloy and Paul Caldwell, *op. cit.*, p. 128.
199. *Ibid.*, p. 69.

CHAPTER 10
200. John Simpson, interview, Cape Town, 18.12.2003.
201. *Ibid.*
202. 'Black Unions: What Danger?', *Sunday Times*, 9 March 1980.
203. Kate Jowell, as quoted in the newsletter of the Cape Society of Chartered Accountants, Autumn 1980, number 8.
204. *Ibid.*
205. *Ibid.*
206. *Ibid.*
207. *Ibid.*
208. Albie Sachs, interview, Cape Town, 30.8.2003.
209. Kate Jowell, as quoted in the newsletter of the Cape Society of Chartered Accountants, *op. cit.*
210. Kate Jowell, as quoted in 'Meat Strike end "victory for no one"', *The Argus*, 8 June 1980.
211. *Ibid.*
212. Naas Steenkamp, interview, Somerset West, 13.10.2005.
213. *Ibid.*
214. Kate Jowell, as quoted in 'Slabbert welcomes PM's tax move', *Weekend Argus*, 19 July 1980.
215. *Ibid.*
216. *Ibid.*

217. Neil Jowell, interview, Cape Town, 5.6.2003.
218. Harris Gordon, interview, Cape Town, 5.6.2003.
219. Robert Rotberg, interview, Johannesburg, 6.6.2003.
220. Gorry Bowes Taylor, 'Clear Tax Line', *Weekend Argus*, 23 October 1980.
221. Sue Garbett, 'A woman's voice on taxation', *Daily News*, 3 November 1980.
222. *Ibid.*
223. As quoted in Sue Garbett, *op. cit.*
224. *Ibid.*
225. *Ibid.*
226. Sue Garbett, 'Inroads into manpower', *The Star*, 5 January 1980.
227. AN Wilson, *Iris Murdoch – As I Knew Her* (London: Hutchinson, 2003), p. 134.
228. Neil Jowell, interview, Cape Town, 16.6.2003.
229. Neil Jowell, interview, Cape Town, 16.6.2003.
230. David Shenk, *op. cit.*, p. 35.
231. *Ibid.*
232. *Ibid.*, p. 36.
233. Alexandra Aleksic, interview, Cape Town, 25.3.2003.
234. *Ibid.*

CHAPTER 11
235. *Illustrated History of South Africa – The Real Story* (South Africa: The Reader's Digest Association Ltd), p. 472.
236. 'The Labour Cause', *The Argus*, 25 May 1981.
237. *Ibid.*
238. *Ibid.*

239. Neil Jowell, interview, Cape Town, 12.3.2003.
240. *Ibid.*
241. *Ibid.*
242. Neil Jowell, interview, Cape Town, 26.5.2003.
243. John Simpson, interview, Cape Town, 18.12.2003.
244. *Ibid.*
245. 'Labour in SA has a long way to go', *Sunday Times*, 19 July 1981.
246. *Ibid.*
247. 'Call for new system of collective bargaining', *Cape Times*, 5 June 1982.
248. *Ibid.*
249. 'Womanpower', *SA Financial Mail*, 2 October 1981.
250. 'Praise for new employment law', *The Star*, 11 February 1983.
251. *Ibid.*
252. Don Lilford, 'Lively debate on tax', *The Argus*, 4 August 1983.

CHAPTER 12

253. Justine Jowell, interview, Cape Town, 21.2.2003.
254. Justine Jowell, interview, Cape Town, 5.3.2004.
255. Kate Jowell, as quoted in 'No Room at the Top? Women and Big Business', *Fair Lady*, 22 August 1984, p. 54.
256. *Ibid.*, p. 53.
257. *Ibid.*
258. *Ibid.*
259. Kate Jowell, as quoted in Linda Vergnani, 'How do women get to the top?', *The Argus*, 24 March 1984.
260. *Ibid.*
261. *Ibid.*

262. 'A Healthy Potential', *Financial Mail* supplement, 16 September 1983.
263. *Ibid.*
264. *Illustrated History of South Africa – The Real Story, op. cit.*, p. 473.
265. *Ibid.*, p. 479.
266. Neil Jowell, interview, Cape Town, 18.5.2006.
267. Kate Jowell, 'Tax: "Women must organize"', *Cape Times*, 7 March 1984.
268. Barend du Plessis, 'Tax overhaul report by mid-1986 – Du Plessis', *Cape Times*, 10 November 1984.
269. Cecil Margo, as quoted in Alec Hogg, 'First Margo report on tax likely in February', *Sunday Times*, 18 November 1984.
270. Jannie Graaff, interview, Cape Town, 10.2.2004.
271. Report of the Commission of Inquiry into the Tax Structure of the RSA, p. 151.
272. 'University of Cape Town – a survey', *Financial Mail* supplement, 1 June 1984.
273. *Ibid.*
274. Paul Bowman, interview, Cape Town, 12.7.2003.
275. *Ibid.*

CHAPTER 13

276. Kate Jowell, interview, Cape Town, 9.9.2003.
277. David Shenk, *op. cit.*, p. 117.
278. *Ibid.*
279. *Ibid.*, p. 126.
280. *Ibid.*

281. Neil Jowell, interview, Cape Town, 8.9.2003.
282. As quoted in Godfrey de Bruyn, 'Kate Jowell – Informed and Perceptive', *Sun*, January 1987, p. 12.
283. Kate Jowell, as quoted in Sheryl Raine, 'Cosatu divided over tactics, says labour expert', *The Star*, 5 September 1986.
284. Kate Jowell, as quoted in Alan Fine, 'Bosses urged to join unions in the search for solutions', *Business Day*, 24 October 1986.
285. Kate Jowell, as quoted in Maggie Rowley, 'Talk with unions, bosses urged', *The Argus*, 14 May 1987.
286. As quoted in Robyn Rafel, 'Under Siege', *Finance Week*, 14–20 May 1987.
287. Kate Jowell, as quoted in Maggie Rowley, *op. cit.*
288. As quoted in Michael Morris, *Every Step of the Way – The Journey to Freedom in South Africa* (Cape Town: HSRC Press, 2004), p. 238.
289. As quoted in Audrey D'Angelo, 'Overseas verdict crucial', *Cape Times*, 9 May 1987.
290. Mike Page, interview, Cape Town, 24.4.2003.
291. Paul Bowman, interview, Cape Town, 22.4.2004.
292. Kate Jowell, interview, Cape Town, 6.1.2003.
293. Kate Jowell, interview, Cape Town, 31.1.2003.
294. Neil Jowell, interview, Cape Town, 8.9.2003.
295. Neil Jowell, interview, Cape Town, 11.7.2006.
296. Phyllis Jowell, *op. cit.*, p. 167.
297. *Ibid.*
298. *Ibid.*, p. 292.
299. Neil Jowell, interview, 8.9.2003.
300. As quoted in Roger Williams, 'Transport man wins our award for business', *Cape Times*, 18 November 1987.
301. Audrey D'Angelo, 'Trencor: One of the JSE's star performers', *Cape Times*, 18 November 1987.
302. *Ibid.*
303. Neil Jowell, as quoted in Audrey D'Angelo, *op. cit.*
304. Zelda Gordon-Fish, *op. cit.*, p. 58.
305. *Ibid.*
306. *Ibid.*
307. *Ibid.*, p. 64.

CHAPTER 14
308. David Shenk, *op. cit.*, p. 87.
309. William Molloy and Paul Caldwell, *op. cit.*, p. 91.
310. Lindy Smit, interview, Glencoe Road, 15.5.2009.
311. William Molloy and Paul Caldwell, *op. cit.*
312. Eunice Mzondi, interview, Cape Town, 5.3.2004.
313. *Ibid.*
314. *Ibid.*
315. Kate Jowell, interview, 31.1.2003.
316. *Ibid.*
317. Nicola Jowell, interview, 11.1.2003.
318. Neil Jowell, interview, 29.5.2009.
319. Nicola Jowell, interview, 11.1.2003.
320. *Ibid.*
321. 'A far from immaculate conception', *University of Cape Town News Special*

Edition: The Graduate School of Business – Twenty Five Years (no date), p. 4.

322. *Ibid.*

323. Ian Gillespie, *ibid.*, p. 6.

324. *University of Cape Town News Special Edition: The Graduate School of Business – Twenty-Five Years, op. cit.*, p. 8.

325. Trevor Williams, telephone interview, 23.4.2003.

326. From The History Channel website, www.historychannel.com.

327. Trevor Williams, telephone interview, 23.4.2003.

328. *Ibid.*

329. John Simpson, interview, Cape Town, 18.12.2003.

330. *Ibid.*

331. *Ibid.*

332. *University of Cape Town News Special Edition: The Graduate School of Business – Twenty-Five Years, op. cit.*, p. 9.

333. *Ibid.*, p. 11.

334. *Ibid.*, p. 10.

335. *Ibid.*, p 9.

336. *Ibid.*

337. Mike Page, interview, Cape Town, 24.4.2003.

338. *Ibid.*

339. *University of Cape Town News Special Edition: The Graduate School of Business – Twenty-Five Years, op. cit.*, p. 9.

340. Jannie Graaff, interview, Cape Town, 10.2.2004.

341. *Ibid.*

342. Mike Page, interview, Cape Town, 24.4.2003.

343. John Simpson, interview, Cape Town, 18.12.2003.

344. Trevor Williams, telephone interview, 23.4.2003.

345. Mike Page, interview, Cape Town, 22.4.2003.

346. John Simpson, interview, 24.4.2003.

347. As quoted in Gorry Bowes Taylor, 'Business brains where once prisoners trod', *Weekend Argus*, 5 September 1992.

348. *Reader's Digest Illustrated History of South Africa – The Real Story* (Cape Town: The Reader's Digest Association, 1994), p. 481.

349. As quoted in Gorry Bowes Taylor, 'Business brains where once prisoners trod', *op. cit.*

350. *Ibid.*

351. *Ibid.*

352. From Academy of Achievement website www.achievement.org and Forbes website www.Forbes.com.

353. Mike Page, interview, Cape Town, 22.4.2003.

354. Trevor Williams, telephone interview, 23.4.2003.

355. Justine Jowell, interview, Cape Town, 21.2.2003.

356. Justine Jowell, interview, Cape Town, 21.2.2003.

357. Neil Jowell, interview, Cape Town, 8.9.2003.

358. *Ibid.*

359. *Ibid.*

360. *Ibid.*

CHAPTER 15

361. The Breakwater Lodge website, www.bwl.co.za.

362. Norman Faull, interview, Cape Town, 8.9.2005.

363. Frank Horwitz, interview, Cape Town, 14.9.2005.

364. As quoted in Zelda Gordon-Fish, 'The Director's Chair', *op. cit.*, p. 64.

365. Norman Faull, interview, 8.9.2005.

366. Kate Jowell, as quoted in Alide Dasnois, 'Kate Jowell – ready and getting down to business', *Weekend Argus*, 6 February 1993.

367. *Ibid.*

368. Norman Faull, interview, Cape Town, 8.9.2005.

369. Mike Page, interview, Cape Town, 22.4.2003.

370. As quoted in *UCT News*, May 1993.

371. Yvonne van Stolk, telephone interview, 20.3.2003.

372. *Ibid.*

373. Frank Horwitz, interview, Cape Town, 14.9.2005.

374. Michael Morris, *op. cit.*, p. 259.

375. As quoted in Audrey D'Angelo, 'GSB gears up to widen management talent pool', *Business Report*, 15 February 1993.

376. *Ibid.*

377. *Ibid.*

378. As quoted in Fred Roffey and Jeremy Woods, 'Campus at the top of Africa's business map', *Sunday Times Business Times*, 29 May 1994.

379. *Ibid.*

380. As quoted in 'GSB is tops in South Africa' (date and publication not supplied).

381. As quoted in Alan Duggan, 'Business School anticipates boom year', *Sunday Times Metro*, 12 January 1997.

382. University of Cape Town official website. www.uct.ac.za.

383. Frank Horwitz, interview, Cape Town, 14.9.2005.

384. *Ibid.*

385. Professor Robert Rotberg directs the Program on Intrastate Conflict and Conflict Resolution at Harvard University's Kennedy School of Government. He first met Kate Jowell in 1980 at the Massachusetts Institute of Technology, where Kate was a visiting fellow of the Sloan School of Management.

386. Bob Rotberg, interview, Johannesburg, 6.6.2003.

387. Neil Jowell, interview, 12.8.2006.

388. Radio interview on SAFM, *Woman Today*, with Hilary Reynolds.

389. *Ibid.*

390. John Simpson, interview, 18.12.2003.

391. *Ibid.*

392. Radio interview, *Woman Today*, February 1993.

393. Zelda Gordon-Fish, *op. cit.*, p. 56.

394. Justine Jowell, interview, Cape Town, 21.2.2003.

395. *Ibid.*

396. Nicola Jowell, email interview, 29.9.2004.

397. *Ibid.*

398. Justine Jowell, interview, Cape Town, 21.2.2003.

399. William Molloy and Paul Caldwell, *op. cit.*, p. 66.

400. Dhaya Pillay, telephone interview, Johannesburg, 30.1.2003.

401. Mike Page, interview, 24.3.2003.
402. Norman Faull, interview, 8.9.2005.
403. John Simpson, interview, 18.12.2003.
404. Linda Fasham, interview, 21.10.2005.
405. Norman Faull, interview, 8.9.2005.
406. Robert Rotberg, telephone interview, Johannesburg, 6.6.2003.
407. Mike Page, interview, 24.3.2003.
408. Norman Faull, interview, Cape Town, 8.9.2005.

CHAPTER 16
409. Nicola Jowell, telephone interview, Bristol, 18.3.2003.
410. Justine Jowell, interview, Cape Town, 21.2.2003.
411. Nicola Jowell, interview, Cape Town, 11.1.2003.
412. *Ibid.*
413. Eunice Mzondi, interview, Cape Town, 5.3.2003.

414. Nicola Jowell, interview, Cape Town, 11.1.2003.
415. Sue Miller, *The Story of My Father* (New York: Alfred A. Knopf, 2003), p. 156.
416. Paul Bowman, interview, Cape Town, 29.10.2003.
417. Ken McKenzie via email, 25.1.2006.
418. Ken McKenzie, email interview, 1.2.2006.
419. Justine Jowell, email interview, 30.6.2009.
420. Lindy Smit, interview, Cape Town, 2.3.2009.
421. *Ibid.*
422. Neil Jowell, interview, Cape Town, 29.7.2009.
423. Sue Miller, *op. cit.*, p. 165.

EPILOGUE
424. AN Wilson, *op. cit.*, p. 264.